MW01026412

FAMILY EMERGENT/URGENT AND AMBULATORY CARE

THE POCKET NP

Sheila Sanning Shea, MSN, RN, ANP, CEN, is an emergency nurse practitioner (ENP) with over 30 years of clinical experience. She works in the Department of Emergency Medicine at St. Mary Medical Center in Long Beach, California. Ms. Shea established a emergency clinical fellowship for nurse practitioners and physician assistants that includes both didactic and clinical experiences. Ms. Shea is widely published and is an author and reviewer for the *Advanced Emergency Nursing Journal*, and was a contributing author to the *Emergency Nurses Core Curriculum* and *Certified Emergency Nurse Review*. Ms. Shea has taught NPs locally and nationally on a variety of emergent and urgent care topics.

Karen "Sue" Hoyt, PhD, RN, FNP-BC, CEN, FAEN, FAANP, FAAN, is an emergency nurse practitioner (ENP) and works at St. Mary Medical Center in Long Beach, California. She is currently a clinical professor for the NP/DNP programs at the Hahn School of Nursing and Health Science at the University of San Diego. Dr. Hoyt has several peer-reviewed books and publications on clinical practice, research, and management/leadership topics. In 2006, she established the first *Advanced Emergency Nursing Journal*. She conceptualized and has implemented a 2-day course for training ENPs and a train-the-trainer course for NP faculty. She has taught minor procedures workshops for NPs/PAs across the country. As a consultant and educator, she has also written ENP continuing education programs. Dr. Hoyt spearheaded *The Delphi Study on Competencies for NPs in Emergency Care*.

FAMILY EMERGENT/URGENT AND AMBULATORY CARE

THE POCKET NP

Sheila Sanning Shea, MSN, RN, ANP, CEN
Karen "Sue" Hoyt, PhD, RN, FNP-BC, CEN, FAEN, FAANP, FAAN

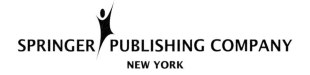

SPRINGER PUBLISHING COMPANY
NEW YORK

Copyright © 2016 Springer Publishing Company, LLC

All rights reserved.

No part of this publication may be reproduced, stored in a retrieval system, or transmitted in any form or by any means, electronic, mechanical, photocopying, recording, or otherwise, without the prior permission of Springer Publishing Company, LLC, or authorization through payment of the appropriate fees to the Copyright Clearance Center, Inc., 222 Rosewood Drive, Danvers, MA 01923, 978-750-8400, fax 978-646-8600, info@copyright.com or on the Web at www.copyright.com.

Springer Publishing Company, LLC
11 West 42nd Street
New York, NY 10036
www.springerpub.com

Acquisitions Editor: Elizabeth Nieginski
Composition: diacriTech

ISBN: 978-0-8261-3413-4
e-book ISBN: 978-0-8261-3414-1

19 20 / 11 10

The author and the publisher of this Work have made every effort to use sources believed to be reliable to provide information that is accurate and compatible with the standards generally accepted at the time of publication. Because medical science is continually advancing, our knowledge base continues to expand. Therefore, as new information becomes available, changes in procedures become necessary. We recommend that the reader always consult current research and specific institutional policies before performing any clinical procedure. The author and publisher shall not be liable for any special, consequential, or exemplary damages resulting, in whole or in part, from the readers' use of, or reliance on, the information contained in this book. The publisher has no responsibility for the persistence or accuracy of URLs for external or third-party Internet websites referred to in this publication and does not guarantee that any content on such websites is, or will remain, accurate or appropriate.

Library of Congress Cataloging-in-Publication Data
Names: Shea, Sheila Sanning, author. | Hoyt, K. Sue, author.
Title: Family emergent/urgent and ambulatory care : pocket np / Sheila
  Sanning Shea, MSN, RN, ANP, CEN, Karen "Sue" Hoyt, PhD, RN, FNP-BC, CEN, FAEN,
  FAANP, FAAN.
Description: New York, NY : Springer Publishing Company, LLC, [2016] |
  Includes bibliographical references and index.
Identifiers: LCCN 2015041188 | ISBN 9780826134134
Subjects: LCSH: Emergency medicine—Handbooks, manuals, etc. | Assistance in emergencies—
Handbooks, manuals, etc. | First aid in illness and injury—Handbooks, manuals, etc.
Classification: LCC RC86 .S54 2016 | DDC 616.02/5—dc23 LC record available at
http://lccn.loc.gov/2015041188

Special discounts on bulk quantities of our books are available to corporations, professional associations, pharmaceutical companies, health care organizations, and other qualifying groups. If you are interested in a custom book, including chapters from more than one of our titles, we can provide that service as well.

For details, please contact:
Special Sales Department, Springer Publishing Company, LLC
11 West 42nd Street, 15th Floor, New York, NY 10036-8002
Phone: 877-687-7476 or 212-431-4370; Fax: 212-941-7842
E-mail: sales@springerpub.com

Printed in the United States of America by Publishers' Graphics.

CONTENTS

PREFACE

Family Emergent/Urgent and Ambulatory Care: The Pocket NP is the result of two decades of our experiences as ENPs. We often found our pockets filled with scribbled notes that included tidbits of things—"Don't Miss!" items and important "Tips" and essential information to include in the history and physical documentation. Although we had many excellent medical reference textbooks, we identified the need for a quick reference guide that had an easy-to-use framework for the most commonly encountered problems seen in the emergency, medical screening, fast-track, and/or primary care setting.

The guide is arranged in a logical head-to-toe format that includes the history and physical examination, and essential medical decision-making considerations. Templates for "Dictation/Documentation" are provided to assist the clinician with the development of a concise and logical patient record. Also included are frequently used illustrations for anatomical reference.

HOW TO USE THIS GUIDE

Use appropriate sections of the "Adult Trauma" or "Adult Medical" templates or "Pediatric" template defaults to document basic normal findings. Delete any portion of the template that was not examined or not pertinent to a specific patient. Mix and match portions of various templates to meet your needs and the components of the physical exam.

Fine-tune your assessment skills using the specific dictation/documentation templates for focused patient problems such as "knee pain."

Demonstrate your critical thinking skills by expanding and polishing your "Medical Decision Making."

"Dictation/Documentation Guidelines" are designed as an outline to ensure that all critical elements of the patient record are addressed.

This guide is just that—a guide. It is intended as a quick reference tool only and it is not meant to be a complete review or definitive guide to clinical practice and patient management. The management options are based on current evidence for best practice. However, emergency medicine is an ever-changing specialty and the user of this guide is encouraged to consult other sources to confirm all medication indications, contraindications, side effects, and dosing prior to administration. The authors and publisher specifically disclaim any liability for errors or omissions found here within or for any misuse or treatment errors.

Sheila Sanning Shea, MSN, RN, ANP, CEN
Karen "Sue" Hoyt, PhD, RN, FNP-BC, CEN, FAEN, FAANP, FAAN

NP SURVIVAL INFORMATION

IMPORTANT PHONE NUMBERS

Main Hospital	
Direct ED	
Fast Track	
Radiology/CT	
Laboratory	
Pharmacy	

COMPUTER ACCESS

Computer ID	
Password	
Computer ID	
Password	
Radiology	
Password	
Transcription	
Password	

NOTES

ABBREVIATIONS*

AAA	Abdominal aortic aneurysm	CVAT	Costovertebral angle tenderness
AB	Abortion	CVD	Cerebrovascular disease
ABC	Airway, breathing, circulation	Cx	culture
ABG	Arterial blood gas	CXR	Chest x-ray
ABO	Blood type groups	D&C	Dilation & curettage
ABX	Antibiotics	D/C	Diarrhea/constipation
ACE	Angiotensin-converting enzyme	DDx	Differential diagnosis
ACI	Aftercare instructions	DIC	Disseminated intravascular coagulopathy
ACS	Acute coronary syndrome	DIP	Distal interphalangeal
AECB	Acute exacerbation chronic bronchitis	DJD	Degenerative joint disease
AGE	Acute gastroenteritis	DM	Diabetes mellitus
ALOC	Altered level of consciousness	DS	Double strength
AMA	Against medical advice	DSD	Dry sterile dressing
AMS	Altered mental status	DTRs	Deep tendon reflexes
A&O	Alert and oriented	DXs	Diagnoses
AP	Anteroposterior	ED	Emergency department
ANUG	Acute necrotizing ulcerative gingivitis	EDC	Estimated date of confinement
APD	Afferent pupillary defect	EDH	Epidural hematoma
ATFL	Anterior talofibular ligament	EKG	Electrocardiogram
AVN	Avascular necrosis	EOMI	Extraocular movements intact
B-hCG	Beta human chorionic gonadotropin	ESR	Erythrocyte sedimentation rate
BID	Twice a day	ETOH	Ethanol
BO	Bowel obstruction	FB	Foreign body
BNP	B-type natriuretic peptide	F/C	Fever/chills
BPV	Benign positional vertigo	FDP	Flexor digitorum profundus
BSA	Bowel sounds active	FDS	Flexor digitorum superficialis
BUN	Blood/urea/nitrogen	FH	Family history
CA	Cancer	FHC	Fitz-Hugh–Curtis syndrome
CAD	Coronary artery disease	FHM	Fetal heart motion/movement
CBC	Complete blood count	FHTs	Fetal heart tones
CCR	Canadian C-spine rules	FOOSH	Fall on outstretched hand
CFL	Collateral fibular ligament	FROM	Full range of motion
CHF	Congestive heart failure	FSBS	Finger stick blood sugar
C/M/S	Circulation/motor/sensation	FTC	Full to confrontation
CMT	Cervical motion tenderness	FX	Fracture
CN	Cranial nerve	G	Gravida
C/O	Complains of	GC	Gonococcal/gonorrhea
COPD	Chronic obstructive pulmonary disease	GCS	Glasgow coma scale
		GERD	Gastroesophageal reflux disease
CP	Chest pain	GI	Gastrointestinal
CRF	Chronic renal failure	GSW	Gunshot wound
CRL	Crown rump length	GU	Genitourinary
CRP	C-reactive protein	HA	Headache
CSF	Cerebrospinal fluid	HCG	Human chorionic gonadotropin
CTA	Clear to auscultation	Hct	Hematocrit
CV	Cardiovascular	HCTZ	Hydrochlorothiazide
CVA	Cerebrovascular accident	Heme	Hematologic

*The abbreviations used in this book may not be accepted medical abbreviations.

Hep C	Hepatitis C	MVC	Motor vehicle crash
HHNK	Hyperglycemic hyperosmolar nonketotic coma	NEXUS	National emergency x-radiography utilization study
HIV	Human immunodeficiency virus	NLP	No light perception
		NS	Normal saline
HM	Hand motion	NT	Nontender(ness) or no tenderness
HOB	Head of bed		
HPI	History of present illness	NTG	Nitroglycerin
HSM	Hepatosplenomegaly	N/V	Nausea/vomiting
HSP	Henoch–Schönlein purpura	N/V/D	Nausea/vomiting/diarrhea
HSV	Herpes simplex virus	NWB	No weight bearing
HTN	Hypertension	OB	Occult blood
HX	History	OPHTH	Ophthalmology
HZV	Herpes zoster virus	OTC	Over the counter
IBD	Irritable bowel disease	P	Para
IBS	Irritable bowel syndrome	PALP	Palpation
ICH	Intracranial hemorrhage	PCN	Penicillin
ICU	Intensive care unit	PE	Pulmonary embolus
IF	Inferior rectus	PEx	Physical examination
IM	Intramuscular	PERRLA	Pupils equal round, reactive to light, accommodation
I&D	Incision and drainage		
IO	Inferior oblique	PID	Pelvic inflammatory disease
IOP	Intraocular pressure	PIP	Proximal interphalangeal
IP	Interphalangeal	PMH	Past medical history
ITP	Idiopathic thrombocytopenia purpura	PNA	Pneumonia
		PND	Paroxysmal nocturnal dyspnea
IUD	Intrauterine device		
IV	Intravenous	PO	Per os; by mouth
IVDA	Intravenous drug addict	POC	Products of conception
IVF	In vitro fertilization	Pt/Pts	Patient/Patients
JVD	Jugular venous distension	PT	Point tenderness
LBP	Lower back pain	PTFL	Posterior talofibular ligament
LCL	Lateral collateral ligament	PUD	Peptic ulcer disease
LLQ	Left lower quadrant	PWD	Pink/warm/dry
LMWH	Low molecular weight heparin	QID	Four times/day
LNMP	Last normal menstrual period	Rh	Rhesus factor
LOC	Level of consciousness	RLQ	Right lower quadrant
LP	Lumbar puncture	RMSF	Rocky mountain spotted fever
LR	Lateral rectus	R/O	Rule out
LS	Lumbosacral	ROS	Review of systems
LUQ	Left upper quadrant	RRR	Regular rate and rhythm
MCL	Medial collateral ligament	RUQ	Right upper quadrant
MDM	Medical decision making	SAB	Spontaneous abortion
MI	Myocardial infarction	SAH	Subarachnoid hemorrhage
MMM	Mucous membranes moist	SaO_2	Oxygen saturation of arterial blood pulse oximetry
MOI	Mechanism of injury		
MR	Medial rectus	SBO	Small bowel obstruction
MRA	Magnetic resonance angiography	SCD	Sickle cell disease
		SCFE	Slipped capital femoral epiphysis
MRN	Medical record number		
MRSA	Methicillin-resistant *Staphylococcus aureus*	SCIWORA	Spinal cord injury without radiographic abnormality
		SDH	Subdural hematoma
MSK	Musculoskeletal	SH	Social history
MTPJ	Metatarsal phalangeal joint		

SJS	Stevens–Johnson syndrome
sle	Slit lamp exam
SLE	Systemic lupus erythematosis
SLR	Straight leg raise
SNT	Soft, nontender
SO	Superior oblique
SOB	Shortness of breath
SR	Superior rectus
SSS	Scalded skin syndrome
STI	Sexually transmitted infections
STEMI	ST elevation myocardial infarction
STS	Soft tissue swelling
SXS	Symptoms
Ta	Tonometry applanation
TAB	Therapeutic abortion
TAD	Thoracic aortic dissection
TB	Tuberculosis
T&C	Type & crossmatch
TEN	Toxic epidermal necrolysis
TENS	Transcutaneous electrical nerve stimulation
TID	Three times a day
TMs	Tympanic membranes
TMJ	Temporomandibular joint
TMX/SMP	Trimethoprim/ sulfamethoxazole
TOA	Tubo-ovarian abscess
T&S	Type & screen
TSS	Toxic shock syndrome
TTP	Tender to palpation
TV	Tidal volume
UA	Urinalysis
UCG	Urine chroionic gonadotropin
URI	Upper respiratory infection
UTI	Urinary tract infection
VA	Visual acuity
VF	Visual fields
VS	Vital signs
VSS	Vital signs stable
V/Q	Ventilation/Perfusion
WNL	Within normal limits

DICTATION/DOCUMENTATION GUIDELINES

GENERAL INFO
This is [_____] NP/PA
> Date of Service
> Time of Dictation
> Patient Name, Age, Gender
> Medical Record Number
> PMD Name/None/Unknown/Patient cannot recall

CHIEF COMPLAINT
Brief stated complaint
> Note discrepancy between triage/nursing note and what patient reports

HISTORY OF PRESENT ILLNESS
Who provided history?/Who accompanied patient?/Mode of arrival?
> Onset, timing, duration, quality, severity
> Pertinent positive and negative findings, alleviating, or precipitating factors
> Related complaints such as F/C, N/V, diarrhea/constipation, urgency/dysuria, chest pain/SOB
> Focused ROS
> Review of old records as indicated

PAST MEDICAL HISTORY/MEDS/ALLERGIES/IMMUNIZATIONS: SOCIAL/FAMILY HISTORY/PHYSICAL EXAM
(Use "General Medical," "Adult Trauma," or "Pediatric" template as guide.) Note both patient reported pain scale rating and objective level of distress. VS: interpret if normal or abnormal, SaO_2 interpretation, weight in kilogram
> If dictating or using preprinted defaults, take care to delete portions of exam not actually performed
> Elaborate on focused exam of chief complaint rather than using default
> Include a brief head-to-toe exam on any patient with potential occult injury or loss of consciousness, such as fall, MVC, assault

ED COURSE
Include rechecks, outcome of medications (e.g., pain level after medication administration, adverse reactions), fluids, address abnormal vital signs, any complications
> Labs, radiology, EKG interpretation
> Note consultation with attending MD and include plan of care that was discussed and agreed upon. Note whether patient was seen by attending MD
> Telephone consultations/patient examination discussions with patient, family, other resources with MD

PROCEDURES
What procedures were performed and how did patient tolerate
> Note motor/neurovascular status after any splint placed

MEDICAL DECISION MAKING
Brief recap of patient presentation and ED course
> Differential diagnoses considered; what your thoughts are in terms of likelihood of diagnosis
> Discuss complexity of case and the "brain work" involved

IMPRESSION/PROVISIONAL ED DIAGNOSIS DISPOSITION/PLAN
Discharged home in whose care?
> Aftercare instructions, plan for follow-up, including who, when, where
> Specific information about potential complications and warning signs requiring return to ED
> Admission/transfer

END OF DICTATION
This ends the dictation on "Patient Name." Please electronically send to appropriate physician/ specialist
> Note dictation reference number on patient record

ADULT MEDICAL TEMPLATE

GENERAL
The patient is well developed, well nourished, conscious and coherent, in no distress

VITAL SIGNS
Note VS and interpret as normal or abnormal, pulse and oxygen interpretation, weight in kilograms

SKIN
Warm and dry without rash, good texture and turgor

HEENT
Head: Normocephalic without evidence of trauma
Eyes: Sclera and conjunctivae normal; pupils equal, round, and reactive to light and accommodation; extraocular movements are intact
Ears: Canals are patent. Tympanic membranes are clear
Nose/Face: Without rhinorrhea
Mouth/Throat: Mucous membranes are moist. Posterior pharynx clear without erythema or exudates

NECK
Supple without meningismus or adenopathy. Carotids are equal. Trachea midline. No bruits or JVD

CHEST
Normal AP diameter. Good expansion without retractions. Nontender. Lungs are clear to auscultation, bilaterally with good tidal volume

HEART
Regular rate and rhythm. Tones are normal. No murmur, rub, or gallop heard

ABDOMEN
Soft and nontender without masses, guarding, or rebound. Bowel sounds are active. No hepatosplenomegaly

BACK
Without spinal or CVAT

GU
Normal external genitalia without lesions or masses. No hernia noted

PELVIS
Nontender to palpation and stable to compression

PELVIC
Vaginal vault is clear. Cervical os is closed. Uterus nontender and/or normal size. No cervical motion tenderness. Adnexae nontender without mass

RECTAL
Normal tone. No rectal wall tenderness or mass. Stool is brown and heme negative

EXTREMITIES
Full range of motion. Good strength, bilaterally. No clubbing, cyanosis, or edema. Peripheral pulses are intact. Sensation intact

NEURO
A&O × 4; GCS 15. Cranial nerves II–XII intact. Motor and sensory exam nonfocal. Moves all extremities. Speech clear. Gait normal

ADULT TRAUMA TEMPLATE

GENERAL
The patient is well developed. Awake, alert, and conversant, in no apparent distress

VITAL SIGNS
Note VS and interpret as normal or abnormal, pulse oxygen interpretation, weight in kilograms

SKIN
Warm and dry

HEENT
Head: Normocephalic atraumatic without palpable deformities
Eyes: Pupils equal, round, and reactive to light and accommodation. Extraocular movements intact. No periorbital ecchymosis or step-off
Ears: Canals patent. Tympanic membranes are clear. No Battle's sign. No hemotympanum
Nose/Face: Atraumatic. Facial bones are nontender to palpation and stable with attempts at manipulation
Mouth/Throat: No intraoral trauma. Teeth and mandible are intact

NECK
No midline point tenderness, step-off, or deformity to firm palpation of posterior cervical spine Trachea midline. Carotids equal. No masses. No JVD. Full range of motion of the neck without limitation or pain

CHEST
No surface trauma. Nontender without crepitus or deformity. No palpable subcutaneous air Lungs have good tidal volume, lungs clear to auscultation bilaterally

HEART
Regular rate and rhythm. No murmur, rub, or gallop

ABDOMEN
No abrasions or ecchymosis or surface trauma. No distention. Bowel sounds are active. Nontender to palpation; no guarding, rebound, or rigidity. No masses

BACK
No contusions, ecchymosis, or abrasions are noted. Nontender without step-off or deformity to firm midline palpation. No CVAT or flank ecchymosis

GU
Normal external genitalia with no blood at the meatus. No scrotal swelling or tenderness

PELVIS
Nontender to palpation and stable to compression. Femoral pulses strong and equal

RECTAL
Normal tone. No rectal wall tenderness or mass. Stool is brown and heme negative

EXTREMITIES
No surface trauma. Full range of motion without limitation or pain. Good strength in all extremities. Sensation to light touch intact. All peripheral pulses are intact and equal

NEURO
A&O × 4, GCS 15, CN II–XII intact. Motor and sensory exam nonfocal. Reflexes are symmetric

PEDIATRIC MEDICAL TEMPLATE

GENERAL
The patient is a well-developed, well-nourished child who is awake and active. Interacts appropriately with surroundings and examiner, in no acute distress

VITAL SIGNS
Note VS and interpret as normal or abnormal, SaO_2 interpretation, weight in kilograms

SKIN
Pink, warm, and dry. Normal texture and turgor without rash or cyanosis

HEENT
Head: Normocephalic without evidence of trauma. Fontanel normal (if still open)
Eyes: Moist and bright. Sclera and conjunctivae normal. Pupils are equal, round, and reactive to light and accommodation. Extraocular movements intact
Ears: Canals patent. Tympanic membranes clear. No pre- or postauricular lymphadenopathy or erythema
Nose: Patent without rhinorrhea or nasal flaring
Mouth/Throat: Mucous membranes moist. Posterior pharynx clear without lesions, erythema, or exudates

NECK
Full range of motion. Supple without meningismus or lymphadenopathy

CHEST
No retractions noted; no grunting or stridor. Good tidal volume. Lungs clear to auscultation bilaterally; no wheezes, rales, or rhonchi. SaO_2 [_____]%, which is within normal limits (if 95% or >)

HEART
Regular rate and rhythm. No murmur, rub, or gallop is heard

ABDOMEN
Soft, nondistended. Bowel sounds are active. No apparent tenderness. No masses or organomegaly palpated

BACK
Without spinal or CVAT

GU
Normal external genitalia without rash. No hernia noted

EXTREMITIES
Full range of motion. Good strength bilaterally. Neurovascular intact. No cyanosis or edema

NEURO
Alert, active, and developmentally normal for age. GCS 15. Muscle tone good and equal, bilaterally, no focal neurological findings noted

PEDIATRIC TRAUMA TEMPLATE

GENERAL
The pt is well developed. Awake, alert, and conversant in no apparent distress

VITAL SIGNS
Note VS and interpret as normal or abnormal, pulse ox interpretation, weight in kg

SKIN
Warm and dry

HEENT
Head: normocephalic atraumatic without palpable deformities
Eyes: pupils equal, round, and reactive to light. Extraocular movements intact
No periorbital ecchymosis or step-off
Ears: canals patent. Tympanic membranes are clear. No Battle's sign. No hemotympanum
Nose/Face: atraumatic. There is no septal hematoma. Facial bones are nontender to palpation and stable with attempts at manipulation
Mouth/Throat: no intraoral trauma. Teeth and mandible are intact

NECK
No midline point tenderness, step-off, or deformity to firm palpation of posterior cervical spine. Trachea midline. Carotids equal. No masses. No JVD. Full range of motion of the neck without limitation or pain

CHEST
No surface trauma. Nontender without crepitus or deformity. No palpable subcutaneous air. Lungs have good tidal volume with normal breath sounds bilaterally

HEART
Regular rate and rhythm. Tones are normal and clear

ABDOMEN
No abrasions or ecchymosis or surface trauma. No distention. Nontender to palpation; no guarding, rebound, or rigidity. No masses. Bowel sounds are active

BACK
No contusions, ecchymosis, or abrasions are noted. Nontender without step-off or deformity to firm midline palpation. No CVAT or flank ecchymosis

GU
Normal external genitalia with no blood at the meatus. No scrotal swelling or tenderness

PELVIS
Nontender to palpation and stable to compression. Femoral pulses strong and equal

RECTAL
Normal tone. No rectal wall tenderness or mass. Stool is brown and heme negative

EXTREMITIES
No surface trauma. Full range of motion without limitation or pain. Good strength in all extremities. Sensation to light touch intact. All peripheral pulses are intact and equal

NEURO
A&O × 3, GCS 15–4/6/5, CN II–XII intact. Motor and sensory exam nonfocal. Reflexes are symmetric

REVIEW OF SYSTEMS

The ROS is not the same as the HPI, which addresses pertinent positives and negatives of the chief complaint. The ROS is an "inventory" of organ systems to investigate the patient's general state of health

GENERAL
F/C, myalgias, fatigue, sweats, weight loss

DERM
Rash, lesions, itching

NEURO
HA, dizziness, vertigo, weakness, trouble with speech or balance, seizures

EYE
Blurred/double vision, flashing lights, pain, drainage, glasses/contact lenses

ENT/NECK
Earache, ringing in ears, nasal congestion, nosebleeds, sore throat, hoarseness, difficulty swallowing or drooling, neck pain, stiffness, swollen glands

RESP
SOB, wheezing, pleuritic chest pain, cough/sputum, hemoptysis

CV
Chest pain, palpitations/irregular heartbeat, lightheaded/dizzy, syncope, diaphoresis, exertional dyspnea, paroxysmal nocturnal dyspnea, leg pain/swelling

GI
Abdominal pain, N/V, D/C, loss of appetite, heartburn, hematemesis, melena, jaundice

GU
Dysuria, frequency, urgency, hematuria, flank pain, testicular pain/swelling, penile discharge, vaginal bleeding or discharge, menses

MSK
Joint pain/swelling, back pain

HEME
Bruising or bleeding, anemia, clots, transfusions

ENDOCRINE
Polyuria, polydipsia

PSYCH
Hallucinations, depression, suicidal/homicidal ideation

ALLERGIC/IMMUNIZATIONS
No allergies/immunization status. Documentation guidelines vary depending on each billing situation

BILLING CONSIDERATIONS

Level 1 Problem Focused	Level 2–3 Expanded Problem Focused	Level 4 or 5 Detailed or Comprehensive
Chief complaint	Chief complaint	Chief complaint
HPI: Focused 1–3 elements	HPI: 1–3 elements	HPI: > 4 elements OR status of 3 or more chronic or inactive conditions
PMH: None required	PMH	PMH
FH/SH: None required	FH/SH: None required, include if pertinent	FH/SH: Detailed
ROS: None required	ROS: 1 element	ROS: 2–10 elements
Exam: Focused exam of 1 body area or organ system	Exam: Focused exam of 1 body area or organ system plus related organ system or symptom	Exam: Detailed and comprehensive
MDM: Minimal number of diagnostic or treatment options; Minimal or no data reviewed; Minimal risk complications, morbidity or mortality	MDM: Limited number of diagnostic or treatment options; Limited or no data reviewed; Limited risk complications, morbidity or mortality. (Difference in level 2 or 3 depends on complexity of decision making such as consideration of differential diagnoses.)	MDM: Highly complex and detailed

HPI: location, severity, timing, modifying factors, quality, duration, associated symptoms.
PMH: medications, allergies, surgeries/hospitalizations, major illnesses, immunizations.
FH: near relative health status, specific diseases, hereditary disorders, disease risk.
SH: occupation, educational level, marital status, living arrangements, sexual history, tobacco, ETOH, drugs.
ROS: constitutional symptoms, GU, heme, eyes, MSK, endocrine, CV, neurological, allergic/immunologic, respiratory, psych, GI, skin.

Claims submitted to Medicaid and/or Medicare must adhere to the Centers for Medicare & Medicaid Services Documentation Guidelines for Evaluation and Management Services (CMS). Some providers use these guidelines for all payers, whereas others follow the American Medical Association (AMA). Current Procedural Terminology (CPT) and Evaluation and Management (E/M) codes are for nongovernmental payers. Levels of care range from 1 to 5 and in order to "score" a chart for billing a certain level of care and varying numbers of organ systems must be reviewed.

SKIN RASHES/LESIONS

HX
- Onset, duration, pruritic, burning
- F/C, N/V, mucous membrane involvement, palms/soles involvement
- Swelling of face, eyes, intraoral, trouble swallowing or breathing, wheezing, cough, coryza
- Possible exposure, potential allergens, travel, risk for MRSA, family/friends with similar SXS
- Drugs especially meth use, psych HX potential exposure

PE
- **General:** alert, not toxic appearing
- **VS and SaO$_2$**
- **Skin:** PWD
- Note lesion size, shape, color, texture, location, blanching
- **Type:** macular, papular, plaque, wheal, vesicle, pustule, bullae, cyst, nodule, ulcer, fissure, scale
- **Pattern/Distribution:** localized, diffuse, discrete, linear, confluent, annular, grouped, discrete, confluent, dermatomal, guttate (drop-like), zosteriform, reticular, herpetiform, serpiginous, pedunculi/umbilicus, multiform, morbilliform, scarlatiniform, reticular crusts, exudates, excoriation
- Edema, erythema, induration, or fluctuance
- Nikolsky sign: Nikolsky is a skin finding in which the top layers of the skin slip away from the lower layers when slightly rubbed
- **HEENT:**
  - **Head:** normocephalic, atraumatic, kerion, hair loss
  - **Eyes:** PERRLA, EOMI, sclera and conjunctiva clear, periorbital lesions, STS, or erythema
  - **Ears:** canals and TMs normal, pre- or postauricular lymphadenopathy
  - **Nose:** normal, rhinorrhea. Vesicle at tip of nose (Hutchinson sign) concern for ophthalmic HZV
  - **Face:** symmetric, "slapped cheeks," lesions
  - **Mouth/Throat:** MMM, posterior pharynx clear, mucosal lesions, strawberry tongue, palatine petechiae, vesicles, Koplick spots are characterized as clustered, white lesions on buccal mucosa (opposite lower 1st & 2nd molars) pathognomonic for measles
- **Neck:** supple, FROM, lymphadenopathy or meningismus
- **Chest:** CTA, heart sounds normal
- **Heart:** RRR, no murmur, rub, or gallop
- **Abd:** soft, BSA, NT, HSM
- **Back:** spinal or CVAT
- **Extrems:** moves all extrems well with good strength

SKIN RASHES/LESIONS

MDM/DDx

Erythematous: serious erythematous rashes that cause fever include **TSS** (mucous membranes), **Kawasaki disease** (peds, mucocutaneous, lymph nodes, peeling fingertips, strawberry tongue), or Scarlet fever (sandpaper rash). Positive Nikolsky sign, which may indicate **SSS** (peds) or **TEN** (adults). Also consider "red man syndrome" hypersensitivity reaction to Vancomycin. **Maculopapular:** presence of fever my indicate **viral exanthema, drug reaction,** or **pityriasis** (herald patch). In ill-appearing pts with target lesions consider SJS or **erythema multiforme**. Febrile and ill pts with peripheral erythematous lesions should prompt consideration of **RMSF, syphilis,** or **Lyme disease**. More common and benign etiologies are **scabies, eczema, psoriasis, tinea. Vesicular/Bullous:** Diffuse distribution of vesicles or bullae with fever may indicate **varicella, disseminated GC, smallpox,** or DIC. Localized lesions point to serious **necrotizing fasciitis** or benign viral etiologies (e.g., hand–foot–mouth disease). Afebrile etiologies rashes include **bullous pemphigoid, pemphigus vulgaris, contact dermatitis,** HSV, **burn injury, dyshidrotic eczema. Petechiae or Purpura:** Palpable petechiae or purpura in ill-appearing pts are very serious findings. Consider **meningococcemia, disseminated GC, endocarditis,** RMSF or HSP. Autoimmune disorders may cause similar lesions but the pt usually appears well. Flat, no palpable lesions may indicate **DIC, TTP, ITP.** Vasculitis, inflammation of the blood vessels; can be caused by a wide variety of disorders.

PRIMARY LESIONS

- **Macule:** less than 1 cm (over 1 cm is patch)
- **Papule:** solid raised lesion with distinct borders, less than 1 cm; may be domed, flat-topped, umbilicated
- **Nodule:** raised solid lesion more than 1 cm (mass >1 cm)
- **Plaque:** solid, raised, flat-topped (plateau) lesion >1 cm in diameter
- **Vesicle:** raised lesions less than 1 cm in diameter that are filled with clear fluid
- **Pustule:** circumscribed elevated pustular lesions commonly infected
- **Bullae:** circumscribed fluid-filled lesions that are >1 cm in diameter. Wheal: area of edema in the upper epidermis
- **Burrow:** linear lesions produced by infestation of the skin and formation of tunnels

SKIN RASHES/LESIONS

MANAGEMENT

OTC topical ointments/creams can be used for minor skin infections (e.g., Bacitracin, Neosporin). When early MRSA is suspected Muciprocin (Bactroban 0.2%) applied BID to the affected area is recommended for 7–10 days. For more serious infections, oral, IM, IV abx will be used. Treatment with antibiotics will depend on the microorganism (e.g., antibacterials—Clindamycin or Bactrim or Keflex for strep coverage). (Refer to Antibiogram/Antibiotic policy at facility.) **Pruritus:** identify cause, topical medications such as low dose corticosteroids, hydration, avoid prolonged cold or dry conditions. Moisturizing lotions such as Aquaphor or Dermicil. If systemic medications used for pruritis, be aware of increased fall risk. Oral steroids may be required in severe cases and dermatology referral. **Venous insufficiency:** elevation of extremity with compression socks. Consider an ankle–brachial index before ordering compression socks to rule out peripheral arterial disease as a cause of ulcerated area. Overlying dermatitis can be treated with topical steroids and oral antibiotics if infected. **Bullous pemphigoid:** topical steroids can be used for localized lesions but may need systemic steroids which need to be used cautiously in elders to avoid hyperglycemia, HTN, and negative effect on bone density. Specialist consultation may order immunosuppressive agent such as methotrexate. **Herpes zoster:** for patients who present within 72 hr of onset of rash, systemic antiviral medication may be indicated and help reduce duration, acute pain, and postherpetic neuralgia. Acyclovir 800 mg PO 5 × per day × 10 days or use Valcyclovir or Famcyclovir. Postherpetic neuralgia may respond to topical agents such as lidocaine or capsaicin. Other options include opioids, tricyclic antidepressants, and gabapentin. Elders should receive herpes zoster vaccine, which can help reduce the incidence of the disease and degree of postherpetic neuralgia pain. **Erythematous:** Serious erythematous rashes that cause fever include TSS (mucous membranes), TEN (adults). Also consider "Red Man Syndrome" hypersensitivity reaction to Vancomycin. **Maculopapular:** presence of fever may indicate viral exanthema, drug reaction, or pityriasis (herald patch). In ill appearing pts with target lesions consider SJS or erythema multiforme. Febrile and ill pts with peripheral erythematous lesions should prompt consideration of RMSF, syphilis, or Lyme disease. More common and benign etiologies are scabies, eczema, psoriasis, tinea. **Vesicular/bullous:** diffuse distribution of vesicles or bullae with fever may indicate varicella, disseminated GC, smallpox, or DIC. Localized lesions point to serious necrotizing fasciitis or benign viral etiologies (hand-foot-mouth dx). Afebrile etiologies rashes include bullous pemphigoid, pemphigus vulgaris, contact dermatitis, HSV, burn injury, dyshidrotic eczema. **Actinic keratosis:** superficial, flat papules may be covered with dry skin. **Petechiae or purpura:** palpable petechiae or purpura in ill-appearing pts are very serious findings. Consider meningococcemia, disseminated GC, endocarditis, RMSF, or HSP. Autoimmune disorders may cause similar lesions but the pt usually appears well. Flat, no palpable lesions may indicate DIC, TTP, ITP. Vasculitis, inflammation of the blood vessels can be caused by a wide variety of disorders.

SKIN RASHES/LESIONS

DICTATION/DOCUMENTATION

- VS and Mental Status
- **General State of Skin:** color, temperature, moisture, texture, turgor. Note mucous membrane involvement, blisters, peeling, extensive erythema, presence or absence of purpura/petechiae, or secondary infection. Describe rash or lesions, including location, distribution, configuration
- **ACUTE ANAPHYLACTIC REACTIONS:**
  - **Epinephrine:** If IV route is not indicated, IM route preferable to subq route due to more rapid absorption. Anterolateral thigh is the preferred site in children and adults

    0.2–1 mg SC q5–15min (1:1,000 solution), OR

    0.1–0.25 mg IM or SC (1:10,000 solution) over 5–10 minutes, OR

    0.1–0.25 mg IV at rate of 1–4 mcg/min over 5 minutes
  - **Autoinjector:** 0.3 mg (contents of 1 autoinjector) SC/IM once in anterolateral aspect of the thigh; may repeat dose after 5–15 minutes if symptoms persist
  - **Antihistamines:** Diphendydramine 25–50 mg PO q6–8hr; not to exceed 300 mg/day; 10–50 mg (no more than 100 mg) IV/IM q4–6hr; not to exceed 400 mg/day
  - **Corticosteroids:** for prevention of recurrent reactions 40–60 mg/day PO in single daily dose or divided q12hr for 3–10 days
  - **H2 -blockers:** Cimeitdine, Ranitidine, Famotidine
  - **Inhaled beta agonists:** for bronchospasm (Albuterol 1–2 puffs q4–6h prn). Glucagon may be useful in treating refractory cardiovascular effects in pts taking beta-blockers

◐ TIPS

MEDICATION-RELATED RASHES

- ABX: penicillin, cephalosporins
- Sulfonamides, vancomycin
- Nitrofurantoin
- ASA/NSAIDs
- Barbiturates
- Contrast dyes
- Pain meds with codeine
- Seizure Meds: carbamazepine or valproate
- Complementary and alternative medications: echinacea
- Great Mimicker: Early sxs of syphilis are similar to many other rashes

SKIN RASHES/LESIONS

DON'T MISS!

Ill pts with:
- Hypotension
- Meningococcemia
- TSS
- TEN
- SJS
- DIC
- RMSF
- Petechiae
- Purpura

HEADACHE

HX
- Onset: first HA, sudden onset or change from normal HA; "worst ever," "thunderclap"
- Alleviating factors: light, sound, position, foods
- Duration, quality, radiation, unilateral or bilateral, frequency F/C, N/V
- Vision: blurred, photophobia, diplopia, loss of vision, lines, spots
- Nasal congestion, sinus pain, cough, dental problems
- Decreased or loss of hearing, tinnitus
- Facial or temporal tenderness, facial asymmetry
- Neck pain, stiffness
- Dizziness, fainting, seizure
- Muscle weakness, numbness, tingling, problem with balance or speech
- Worse in morning hours (e.g., carbon monoxide), rash
- LNMP
- Recent trauma, onset after exertion
- PMH: HTN, CVA, cardiac
- FH of HA

PE
- **General:** alert, not toxic appearing
- **VS:** fever
- **Skin:** PWD, rash, petechiae
- **HEENT:**
  - **Head:** trigger point, scalp tenderness
  - **Eyes:** PERRLA, sclera, conjunctiva, corneas, EOM, fundi. Note nystagmus, diplopia, ptosis, tearing, conjunctival infection, IOP if measured
  - **Ears:** canals and TMs
  - **Nose:** drainage, congestion
  - **Face:** sinus tenderness, facial swelling, decreased pulsation or tenderness over temple, TMJ tenderness
  - **Mouth/Throat:** MMM, condition of teeth
- **Neck:** supple, FROM, lymphadenopathy, meningismus
- **Chest:** CTA
- **Abd:** soft, NT
- **Extrems:** moves all extrems with good strength, distal motor/sensory intact, good pulses
- **Neuro:** A&O × 4, GCS 15, CN II–XII, focal neuro deficit, DTRs, pathological reflexes, speech/gait, Romberg, pronator drift, speech clear, gait steady

MDM/DDx
MDM includes benign causes of cephalgia such as **migraine**, **cluster** or **tension headaches**, **sinus** or **dental infection**, **TMJ problems**, or **pseudotumor cerebri**. More serious causes include **meningitis** or **encephalitis**, **giant cell arteritis**, **glaucoma**, **subarachnoid hemorrhage**, **subdural/epidural hematoma**, **intracranial bleed** or **tumor**

HEADACHE

MANAGEMENT

- Minimize visual and auditory stimuli, cold compresses, antiemetic
- IV NS 1 L often helpful
- Analgesia options widely vary. NSAIDs; Chlorperazine 5 to 10 mg IV or promethazine 25 mg IV plus diphenhydramine 25 mg IV; metoclopramide 10 to 20 mg IV; abortive agents such as triptans may be effective; opioid, for example, Dilaudid 1–2 mg IV in severe cases
- Lower cervical intramuscular injection
- Consider other causes of HA, such as structural, infectious or metabolic etiologies
- Imaging not usually needed with HX migraine and normal neuro exam
- Admit for intractable N/V or pain
- Neuro consult as needed

LOWER CERVICAL INTRAMUSCULAR INJECTION PROCEDURE: The pt was placed in a seated position and the posterior seventh cervical vertebrae landmark palpated. Sterile drape and prep was done and injection sites were located 2–3 cm lateral to the spinous process. A 25 or 27 gauge needle was introduced 1–1.5 inches parallel to the top of the shoulder in a posterior to anterior direction. Bupivacaine 1.5 mL was slowly injected into the lower paraspinous muscle. The needle was withdrawn and the area massaged to promote absorption of the medication. DSD was applied. Lung sounds were CTA bilaterally after the procedure and the pt tolerated the procedure well. Pain level was ___/0–10 post procedure.

DICTATION/DOCUMENTATION

- **General:** awake and alert, not toxic appearing
- **VS:** no fever or tachycardia
- **SaO$_2$:** WNL
- **Skin:** PWD, no lesions or rash, no petechiae
- **HEENT:**
  - **Head:** scalp atraumatic, NT, no trigger points
  - **Eyes:** sclera and conjunctiva clear, corneas grossly clear, PERRLA, EOMI, no nystagmus, no ptosis, no photophobia, normal fundoscopic exam, normal visual fields, IOP
  - **Ears:** canals and TMs normal
  - **Nose/Face:** no rhinorrhea, congestion; no frontal or maxillary sinus TTP; no asymmetry
  - **Mouth/Throat:** MMM, no erythema or exudate
- **Neck:** supple, FROM, NT, no lymphadenopathy, no meningismus
- **Chest:** CTA
- **Heart:** RRR, no murmur, rub, or gallop
- **Extrems:** moves all extremities with good strength, normal gait
- **Neuro:** A&O × 4; GCS 15. CN II–XII grossly intact. No focal neurological deficits. Normal muscle strength and tone. Normal DTRs, negative Babinski, normal finger-to-nose coordination or heel-to-shin glide, speech clear, normal gait. Negative Romberg, no pronator drift

HEADACHE

CRANIAL NERVES

I	Olfactory	Sense of smell
II	Optic	Visual acuity, visual fields, fundi
III	Oculomotor	Pupillary function, EOM function of IO, SR, MR, IR
IV	Trochlear	EOM function of SO
V	Trigeminal	Facial sensation to light touch, temperature, facial muscle strength, corneal reflex
VI	Abducens	EOM function of LR
VII	Facial	Symmetry of facial expressions (e.g., smile, frown, wrinkle forehead), taste anterior 2/3 of tongue
VIII	Acoustic	Whisper test, tuning fork lateralization
IX	Glossopharyngeal	Gag reflex, swallow, taste posterior 1/3 of tongue
X	Vagus	Gag reflex, swallow, hoarseness, soft palate sensation
XI	Spinal Accessory	Shoulder shrug and turn head against resistance
XII	Hypoglossal	Tongue symmetry, movement, strength

DON'T MISS!

- Systemic illness, febrile, neck stiffness
- First HA, sudden onset, >50 years
- New headache in immunosuppressed pts
- Focal neurological deficits
- Intractable pain
- Head injury
- Glaucoma
- Giant cell arteritis

DIZZY/WEAK

HX

- Onset, intensity, and duration are important clues
- Positional, exacerbated by movement of neck or head
- False sense of motion: feeling of room spinning or pt spinning
- Feeling off balance, about to fall or faint, lightheaded, disoriented
- Headache, N/V, sweating
- Visual changes, blurred vision, loss of vision
- Loss of hearing/tinnitus, ear pain
- Antalgic or ataxia gait
- Numbness, tingling, focal weakness
- Heavy menses, vomiting blood, or blood in stool, trauma
- Fever, poor fluid intake
- CP/dysrhythmia, SOB, syncope, seizure
- Hypoglycemia
- Illicit drugs/ETOH/smoking
- Medication HX: antihypertensives, antiarrhythmics, antianxiolytics. Situational anxiety/hyperventilation

PE

- **General:** mental status
- **VS and SaO$_2$:** tachycardia, bradycardia, dysrhythmia, orthostatic changes
- **Skin:** pale, cool, moist, hot, flushed
- **HEENT:**
  - **Head:** normocephalic, atraumatic
  - **Eyes:** PERRLA, EOMI, ptosis, nystagmus: horizontal, vertical, rotational; changes with fixed gaze diplopia
  - **Ears:** canals and TMs normal, vesicles, hearing
  - **Nose:** normal
  - **Face:** symmetry, facial droop, sensation to light touch and temperature
  - **Mouth/Throat:** MMM, posterior pharynx clear
- **Neck:** supple, FROM, no lymphadenopathy or meningismus
- **Chest:** CTA
- **Abd:** soft, BSA, NT
- **Back:** spinal or CVAT
- **Extrems:** moves all extremities with good strength, distal motor/sensory intact, good pulses
- **Neuro:** A&O x 4, GCS 15, CN II–XII intact, no focal neuro deficits, normal finger-to-nose or heel-to-shin testing, Romberg neg, no prontator drift, rapid alternating movements. Gait is normal, cautious, wide-based, ataxic, tandem gait with eyes closed

⚙ TIPS

- **True Vertigo:** feeling that environment is rotating or spinning, often associated with nausea
- **Central Vertigo:** brainstem or cerebellum—diplopia, N/V, trouble with speech or swallowing, focal weakness, ataxia or unable to ambulate, sudden spontaneous fall with rapid recovery
- **Peripheral Vertigo:** inner ear or vestibular nerve—awake and alert, N/V, usually able to ambulate, very brief episodes of vertigo associated with rapid head movement, tinnitus or hearing loss, HX migraine, recent URI, or barotrauma

DIZZY/WEAK

MDM/DDx

Diplopia, dysarthria, dysphagia, motor and sensory changes, or syncope are serious findings that may be caused by **brainstem ischemia** or **multiple sclerosis**. Lightheadedness and imbalance on assuming upright posture may be **orthostatic changes** caused by antihypertensive or antiarrhythmic medications. Vertigo lasting minutes to hours with hearing changes and headache is often **migrainous** in origin. Very brief episodes of vertigo associated with rapid head movement suggest **BPV**. Vertigo with hearing loss and recent viral illness may be caused by labyrinthitis; while vertigo for hours, hearing loss and tinnitus, fullness or pressure in ear may be caused by **Meniere's disease.** Longer durations of vertigo, days to weeks, with an abrupt onset and associated with N/V but no auditory or neurological findings suggests **vestibular neuronitis.** Vague "heavy-headedness," lightheadedness, and feeling "off balance" without true vertigo and lack of physical findings may be related to **anxiety** disorders but often require neuro referral to rule out serious causes. Rarely, nonmalignant tumors of the eighth CN (**acoustic neuroma**) can cause dizziness and hearing loss. Sudden, severe weakness/dizziness with chest pain radiating to the back may indicate **MI, ACS, CAD, AAA/TAD, PE.**

MANAGEMENT

- **Central Vertigo:** basic labs, EKG, CT/MRI or CTA, neuro consult
- **Peripheral Vertigo:** meclizine 25 mg QID; antiemetics, HCTZ for Meniere's
- **Weak/Lightheaded/Syncope:** EKG, IV volume replacement, monitor, basic labs of cardiac enzymes, coags, T&S, CT/MRI as indicated; possible cardiac or neuro consult; likely admit

DICTATION/DOCUMENTATION

- **General:** alert and active. Ambulates to treatment area with normal gait
- **VS and SaO$_2$:** normal, no orthostatic changes
- **Skin:** PWD, no pallor
- **HEENT:**
    - **Head:** normocephalic, atraumatic
    - **Eyes:** PERRLA, conjunctivae pink, EOMI, no ptosis or nystagmus
    - **Ears:** canals and TMs normal, no vesicles, hearing normal
    - **Nose:** normal
    - **Face:** no facial asymmetry sensation to light touch and temperature intact and symmetrical
    - **Mouth/Throat:** MMM, normal rise of soft palate, posterior pharynx clear
- **Neck:** supple, FROM, no lymphadenopathy or meningismus
- **Chest:** CTA
- **Heart:** RRR, no murmur, rub, or gallop
- **Abd:** soft, BSA, NT
- **Rectal:** brown stool, OB negative
- **Back:** no spinal or CVAT
- **Extrems:** moves all extrems with good strength, distal motor/sensory intact and symmetrical, good pulses
- **Neuro:** A&O x 4, GCS 15, CN II–XII intact, no focal neuro deficits, normal finger-to-nose or heel-to-shin testing, Romberg neg, no prontator drift, normal rapid alternating movements. Gait is normal, cautious, wide-based, ataxic, tandem gait with eyes closed

ALTERED MENTAL STATUS

HX

- Onset rapid or gradual, duration, timing, previous episodes, baseline
- Fluctuating or progressive SXS
- F/C, poor fluid intake/dehydration
- Hypoglycemia, sweating
- Trauma
- Visual/auditory hallucinations, ingestion/overdose of drugs/ETOH/CO exposure
- Headache, fever, N/V, neck pain or stiffness, dizziness/syncope/vertigo/seizure. Visual changes, blurred vision, loss of vision. Loss of hearing/tinnitus, ear pain
- Changes in speech (dysarthria or aphasia), vision (diplopia), or memory (Mini-cog); CP/dysrhythmia, SOB
- Weakness, tremors, bowel/bladder function, melena
- Renal/Met: DM, DKA/HHNK, CRF, hypo/hypernatremia
- Endo: thyroid, Addison's disease
- Neuro: HA, seizure, CVA, SAH, tremors (e.g., Parkinson's), dementia, numbness, tingling, focal weakness; antalgic or ataxia gait, balance problems, motor/sensory changes.
- Psych: anxiety/hyperventilation
- Immunosuppressed pts: HIV, DM, Hep C, CA, HTN, MI/ACS, CAD, CVD, AAA/TAD, PE, connective tissue disease (e.g., Marfan's syndrome)
- ETOH, illicit drug use, tobacco
- Meds: New or recently changed/stopped meds, OTC, home remedies, antihypertensive, anticoagulants, opioids, antiepileptics

PE

- **General:** alert, disoriented, confused, tremulous, arousable, agitated, lethargic, stuporous, delirious, comatose. Hygiene; trauma; odors (ETOH, acetone, almonds)
- **VS and SaO$_2$:** fever/hypothermia, brady/tachycardia, resp depression, hypo/hyperventilation
- **Skin:** texture, turgor, rash, petechiae/purpura, jaundice, needle marks
- **HEENT:**
  - **Head:** surface trauma
  - **Eyes:** PERRLA, fixed/dilated, icterus, EOMI, ptosis, fundi (papilledema, retinal hemorrhage)
  - **Ears:** canals patent, hemotympanum, CSF leak
  - **Nose:** CSF leak
  - **Face:** symmetric, weakness
  - **Mouth/Throat:** gag reflex, tongue symmetry
- **Neck:** meningismus, nuchal rigidity, thyroid
- **Chest:** CTA, heart RRR, respiratory effort
- **Heart:** RRR or arrhythmias
- **Abd:** soft, NT, pulsatile mass, ascites, hepatomegaly, suprapubic TTP or distension
- **Extrems:** FROM, NT, strength and sensation, weakness, tremors, asterixis (liver hand flap), rigidity
- **Rectal:** tone, occult blood, melena
- **Neuro:** A&O × 4, GCS 15, CN II–XII, focal neuro deficit, DTRs, pathological reflexes, Romberg, pronator drift, speech clear, gait steady, spontaneous or uncontrolled movements, abnormal posturing, flaccid

ALTERED MENTAL STATUS

MDM/DDx

Pts with AMS can range from slightly confused to comatose. A thorough HX and knowledge of pt's baseline is essential. AMS is not a diagnosis and MDM is directed toward identification of underlying cause. Initial MDM is directed at stabilization of ABCs, evaluation for possible surgical intervention and admission. **Hypoxia** and **hypoglycemia**, **opiate ingestion**, **intracranial hemorrhage** are common causes of AMS and easily treated. Head trauma may or not be evident; check pupils, fundoscopic, hemotympanum. Assess for signs of **infection**, such as hypo or hyperthermia and tachycardia, nuccal rigidity, petechiae. Urosepsis and pneumonia are common infections that cause AMS. Immediate ABX if suspicious for **sepsis**. For AMS of **unclear etiology** consider UA/Utox, complete metabolic panel (with Mg/Phos), LFTs, ABG. Also EKG, CXR, CT, and/or LP. Infants, older adults, debilitated, and immunosuppressed are high risk groups. Sudden, severe chest pain radiating to the back may indicate MI/ACS, CAD, **AAA/TAD**, pulmonary embolus (PE).

MANAGEMENT

- Full spinal immobilization if trauma suspected
- ABCs with spinal immobilization if trauma suspected
- O$_2$, IV NS, FSBS, CBC, chem panel, UA, Utox
- Consider: LFTs, ABG, specific drug levels, carboxyhemoglobin
- EKG, CXR, head CT, LP, C-spine x-ray (if trauma)
- Flumazenil, narcan, thiamine

DICTATION/DOCUMENTATION

- **General:** awake and alert, not toxic appearing. No odors. VSS, no fever or tachycardia
- **VS and SaO$_2$**
- **Skin:** PWD, no lesions or rash, no surface trauma noted
- **HEENT:**
    - **Head:** scalp atraumatic, NT
    - **Eyes:** sclera and conjunctiva clear, corneas grossly clear, PERRLA, EOMI, no nystagmus or disconjugate gaze, no ptosis. Corneal reflex intact. Fundoscopic exam
    - **Ears:** canals and TMs normal. No hemotympanum or Battle's sign
    - **Nose/Face:** atraumatic, NT, no asymmetry
    - **Mouth/Throat:** MMM, posterior pharynx clear, normal gag reflex, no intraoral trauma
- **Neck:** supple, FROM, NT, no lymphadenopathy, no meningismus
- **Chest:** CTA, no wheezes, rhonchi, rales. Normal TV, no retractions or accessory muscle use. No respiratory depression
- **Heart:** RRR, no murmur, rub, or gallop
- **Abd:** soft, NT, pulsatile mass, ascites, hepatosplenomegaly, suprapubic TTP, or distension
- **Back:** without spinal or CVA tenderness
- **Extrems:** moves all extremities with good strength, distal motor neurovascular intact
- **Neuro:** A&O × 4, GCS 15, CN II–XII grossly intact. No focal neurological deficits. Normal muscle strength and tone. Normal DTRs, negative Babinski, normal finger-to-nose coordination or heel-to-shin glide. Speech, gait, Romberg neg, no pronator drift

ALTERED MENTAL STATUS

LUMBAR PUNCTURE PROCEDURE NOTE: After obtaining informed consent from the pt/parent, the pt was prepped, draped, and cleansed with povidone–iodine/saline in sterile fashion. Appropriate landmarks were identified and the area was infiltrated with ( ) mL 1% Lidocaine with good surface infiltration. ( ) gauge (22 g for peds) was inserted between L4 and L5. Opening pressure measurement was ( ). Approx ( ) mL of (clear, cloudy, bloody) fluid was obtained. The needle was withdrawn and a dry, sterile dressing was applied. The pt tolerated the procedure well without complications.

TERMS
- **Altered:** nonspecific term
- **Lethargy:** awake but drowsy, listless, depressed LOC
- **Stupor:** rouses to vigorous stimuli
- **Delirium:** transient and/or fluctuating mental confusion
- **Dementia:** gradual, progressive decline in memory, judgment, thinking
- **Coma:** unresponsive to external stimuli

AEIOU TIPS FOR ALTERED MENTAL STATUS

A Alcohol	T Trauma
Alzheimer's	Tumor
E Electrolytes	Toxicology
Endocrine	I Insulin (too much/too little)
Encephalopathy	P Psych
Environmental	Poison
I Infection	S Seizure
O Overdose	Sepsis
U Uremia	Stroke

◯ TIPS
- Never assume psych cause of AMS until medical etiologies excluded
- Look first for readily treatable causes
- Be sure chart reflects attempts to obtain history from pt, others, PMD, medical records
- Be wary of AMS pt leaving AMA

HEAD INJURY

HX
- Time on injury, MOI (auto vs. ped, ejection, significant fall)
- ALOC: gradual, sudden LOC, brief lucid interval
- HA, visual changes, seizure
- Blood/CSF leak nose/ears
- Neck/back pain, N/V
- Age >60, use of anticoags, ETOH
- Distracting injury, suspected open or depressed skull FX

PEDS
- Concern for basilar skull FX, skull penetration
- Large scalp hematoma
- Fall >3 ft or > 5 steps or > 3 × child's height
- ALOC, irritable, lethargic
- Serious MVC, unrestrained, auto vs. ped

PE
- **General:** position of pt (full spinal precautions)
- **VS and SaO$_2$:** tachycardia or bradycardia (significant for shock/neurogenic shock), widening pulse pressure
- **Skin:** warm, dry, cool, moist, pale
- **HEENT:**
  - **Head:** surface trauma, TTP, bony step-off
  - **Eyes:** PERRLA, EOMI, periorbital ecchymosis
  - **Ears:** canals patent, TMs, Battle's sign, hemotympanum, CSF leak
  - **Nose:** nasal injury, septal hematoma, epistaxis, CSF rhinorrhea
  - **Face:** facial trauma
  - **Mouth/Throat:** intraoral trauma, teeth and mandible stable
- **Neck:** FROM without limitation or pain, NT to firm palp at midline
- **Chest:** NT, CTA
- **Heart:** RRR, no murmur, rub, or gallop, clear tones
- **Abd:** soft, BSA, NT
- **Back:** no spinal or CVAT
- **Pelvis:** NT to palpation and stable to compression, femoral pulses strong and equal
- **Extrems:** FROM, NT, distal CMS intact
- **Neuro:** A&O × 4, GCS 15, no focal neuro deficits

CONCUSSION ASSESSMENT CRITERIA:
Recall of person, place, time, events?
Five simple word recall
Months of year in reverse order
Random 3 to 6 numbers in reverse: if able to recall three digits correctly in reverse order, increase number of digits in sequence; speech, pupils, EOMs, gait

Adapted from McCroy, P., Johnson, K., Meeuwisse, W., Aubry, M., Cantu, R., Dvorak, J., … Schamasch, P. (2005). Summary and agreement statement of the 2nd International Conference on Concussion in Sport, Prague 2004. *British Journal of Sports Medicine, 39*(4), 196–204.

HEAD INJURY

MDM/DDx

Differential diagnoses considered include **mild blunt head injury** and/or **scalp laceration**. Serious problems include **concussion**, **skull fracture**, **subdural** or **epidural hematoma**, **cerebral contusion**, and **intracranial hemorrhage**. MDM must consider those pts with **high risk** for significant injury, drug/ETOH use, distracting injuries, or anticoagulant use. Also, age >60 years, suspected open or depressed skull FX, evidence of basilar skull FX (periorbital ecchymosis, hemotympanum, Battle's sign, CSF leak), vomiting, GCS < 15 at 2 hours postinjury, deteriorating during observation, or postinjury amnesia > 2 to 4 hrs. Consider **predictable injury** based on mechanism such as fall > 3 ft or five stairs, ejection from vehicle, auto vs. pedestrian.

MANAGEMENT

- Mild injury with low risk may be observed and given analgesia and antiemetic as needed; good ACI and close follow-up. Persistent N/V, severe headache, amnesia, LOC, or intoxication require head CT and observation of several hours before decision to discharge. Consult neuro for abnormal CT findings or not stable for discharge.

DICTATION/DOCUMENTATION

- **General:** awake and alert in no distress; no odor of ETOH
- **VS and SaO$_2$**
- **Skin:** PWD, no surface trauma
- **HEENT:**
  - **Head:** atraumatic, no palpable deformities. Fontanele flat (if still open)
  - **Eyes:** PERRLA, EOMI, no periorbital ecchymosis
  - **Ears:** TMs clear, no hemotympanum or Battle's sign
  - **Nose/Face:** atraumatic. No septal hematoma. Facial bones symmetric, NT to palpation and stable with attempts at manipulation
  - **Mouth/Throat:** no intraoral trauma. Teeth and mandible are intact
- **Neck:** no point tenderness, step-off or deformity to firm palpation of the cervical spine at the midline. No spasm or paraspinal muscle tenderness. Trachea midline. Carotids equal. FROM without limitation or pain
- **Chest:** no surface trauma or asymmetry. NT without crepitus or deformity. Normal tidal volume. CTA bilaterally. Oxygen saturation greater than 95% on room air
- **Heart:** RRR, no murmur, rub, or gallop. All peripheral pulses are intact and equal.
- **Abd:** nondistended without abrasions or ecchymosis. Bowel sounds are active. NT, guarding or rebound. No masses. Good femoral pulses
- **Back:** no contusions, ecchymosis, or abrasions are noted. NT without step-off or deformity to firm palpation of the thoracic and lumbar spine
- **Pelvis:** NT to palpation and stable to compression
- **GU:** normal external genitalia, no blood at the meatus (if applicable)
- **Rectal:** normal tone. No rectal wall tenderness or mass. Stool is brown and heme negative (if applicable)
- **Extrems:** no surface trauma. FROM. Distal motor, neurovascular supply is intact.
- **Neuro:** A&O × 4, GCS 15, CN II–XII grossly intact. Motor and sensory exam nonfocal. Reflexes are symmetric. Speech is clear and gait steady

EYE PAIN

HX

- Baseline vision, previous HA or eye problems, surgeries. Corrective glasses, contacts, or protective eyewear. Onset, duration, unilateral, or bilateral
- Visual changes: FB sensation, photophobia, diplopia, decreased or loss of vision, flashes of lights, halos, veil, or curtain, scotoma (area of loss of vision surrounded by normal vision). Transient monocular blindness consider AAA/TAD
- Redness, discharge, tearing, itching, burning, swelling
- Painful or restricted eyeball movement
- Nasal congestion, sinus pain, cough
- Facial lesions, redness, swelling
- F/C, N/V, rash, genital lesions
- MOI: grinding metal or FB under pressure, chemical exposure, organic matter injury, blunt or penetrating trauma
- Comorbidities: HAs, migraines, DM, CAD, CA, HTN, glaucoma, herpes, sinus problems; work related, day care, sick contacts

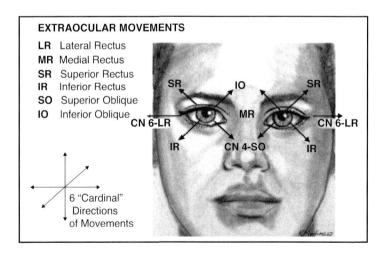

EXTRAOCULAR MOVEMENTS

LR Lateral Rectus
MR Medial Rectus
SR Superior Rectus
IR Inferior Rectus
SO Superior Oblique
IO Inferior Oblique

SR   IO   SR
CN 6-LR   MR   CN 6-LR
IR   CN 4-SO   IR

6 "Cardinal"
Directions
of Movements

EYE PAIN

PE

- **General:** level of distress
- **VS and SaO$_2$**
- **Skin:** warm, dry, cool, moist, pale
- **HEENT:**
    - **Head:** surface trauma, TTP, bony step-off
    - **Eyes: Visual Acuity (V$_A$):** Snellen chart, count fingers (CF), hand motion, light or shadow or NLP
    - **Visual Fields (V$_F$):** FTC
    - **Periorbital:** STS, erythema, warmth, tenderness, bony step-off, or deformity
    - **Eyelids:** erythema, crusting, swelling, FB/lesion on lid eversion, elevation (CN 3); closure (CN 7)
    - **Eyeballs:** enophthalmos or exophthalmos, tenderness, intact
    - **Pupils:** PERRLA; CN 2 senses incoming light (afferent); CN 3 constricts pupil (efferent)
    - **Corneas:** grossly clear, steamy, no obvious FB or hyphema/hypopyon
    - **Sclera:** clear, injected, ciliary or limbic flush
- **Neuro:** exam as indicated
- **Conjunctiva:** palpebral and bulbar, subconjunctival hemorrhage, chemosis, evert lids
- **EOMI:** symmetry of gaze, limitation or pain, nystagmus, ptosis, lid lag
- **Lacrimal System:** canthus, papilla, puncta
- **Fundoscopic Exam:** retina
- **APD:** abnormal constriction due to unilateral afferent pathway problem
- **Fluorescein Stain Exam:** corneal epithelial defect, abrasion, ulcer, dendritic lesion, FB, rust ring
- **Slit Lamp Exam:** anterior chamber clear or cell/flare, hyphema, hypopyon; tonometry measurement of IOP normal < 20
- **Ears:** canals and TMs, lesions
- **Nose/Face:** drainage, congestion; TTP, erythema, decreased pulsation of temporal artery, erythema, warmth, tenderness, bony step-off, or deformity
- **Mouth/Throat:** MMM, posterior pharynx
- **Neck:** supple, lymphadenopathy, meningismus

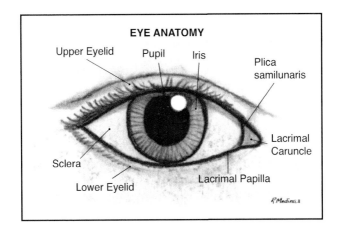

EYE ANATOMY

Upper Eyelid
Pupil
Iris
Plica samilunaris
Lacrimal Caruncle
Lacrimal Papilla
Sclera
Lower Eyelid

EYE PAIN

MDM/DDx

Eye pain is a frequent complaint of ED pts and can be divided into either ocular or orbital in nature. Ocular eye problems involve the structures of the surface of the eye and range from benign to vision threatening problems. **Conjunctivitis** may be allergic, viral, bacterial, fungal, or chemical and can progress to involve the cornea (**keratitis** or **keratoconjunctivitis**), which may look like stippling or punctuate lesion. FBs under the upper lid or embedded in the cornea are a common problem; **metallic FBs** can cause a rust ring and result in visual defects. Damage to the corneal epithelium leads to painful corneal abrasions that fluoresce under cobalt light. Fluorescein stain can also identify **dendritic lesions** caused by **HSV**. **HZV** can cause a pseudodendrite and may be associated with facial **HZV** lesions; **Hutchinson's sign** is an HZV lesion on the tip of the nose that has a high correlation to involvement of the eye. Severe pain, tearing, blurred vision, and focal whitish infiltrate in stromal layer indicate a **corneal ulcer**, which is a common complication of **contact lens** use. This ophthalmologic emergency can lead to permanent visual damage and/or perforation. **Periorbital infections** include infections of the soft tissues or lacrimal system. Periorbital cellulitis (referred to as preseptal) involves the area anterior to the orbital septum, which acts as a barrier to the actual eyeball. The area is swollen, erythematous, and warm but movement of the EOMs is unlimited and painless, and there is no proptosis. **Dacryocystitis** is an inflammation of the lacrimal duct or sac while **dacryoadenitis** involves the lacrimal gland in the supraorbital area. **Orbital cellulitis** results when infection has spread to the eyeball itself. The pt appears ill with fever, visual changes, headache, and restricted and painful movement of the eye. Proptosis and possible meningeal signs. **Orbital pain** results from eyeball disease or trauma and causes a deep ache in or behind the eye. Deeper structure problems include iritis and **uveitis** and are characterized by severe pain unrelieved by topical anesthesia, tearing, and ciliary or limbic flush. SLE will usually reveal cells and flare from inflammation. N/V and HA are common complaints of pts with a painful red eye caused by **acute narrow-angle glaucoma** and require immediate consultation. Complaints of **loss of vision** without pain ("quiet eye") suggest **detached retina**, **central retinal artery occlusion**, **complete hyphema**, **vitreous hemorrhage**, or **optic neuritis**. FBs may enter the eye and lodge in the intraocular space. Assess for globe integrity if penetrating trauma is suspected. Signs of **globe disruption** can be subtle, such as Seidel sign (leakage of fluorescein stain), or obvious visible vitreous humor. Eye pain can also be related to sinus or dental problems, or migraine HA.

EYE PAIN

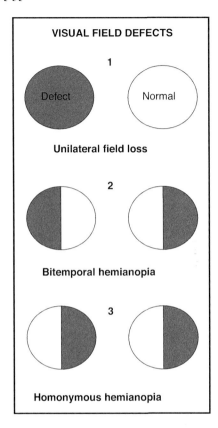

VISUAL FIELDS
- **Unilateral Blindness:** (amarosis fugax) transient loss of vision; TIA, optic neuritis, temporal arteritis
- **Bitemporal Hemianopsia:** blindness of temporal or outer fields of both eyes; tumor
- **Homonymous Hemianopsia:** optic tract problem causing blindness in temporal or nasal field of one or both eyes; stroke

APD "SWINGING LIGHT TEST": Tests for light being "sensed" and needs intact pathway of globe, retina, optic nerve. In dark room, shine light into one eye; swing quickly to other, then back and forth. Normally, both pupils constrict equally without redilation. Affected pupil will not constrict if light not "sensed" but constricts when stimulated by light directed into normal eye, then dilates. Most common pupillary defect. Hyphema or vitreous hemorrhage will not cause APD.

EYE PAIN

MANAGEMENT

- **Conjunctivitis/Keratitis:** usually viral, supportive care
- **Bacterial:** polymyxin B/trimethoprim 1 to 2 gtts every 3 to 6 hours × 7 to 10 days; erythromycin oint ½" QID; levofloxacin 0.5% 1 to 2 gtts every 2 hours while awake × 2 days, then QID × 5 days; tobramycin 0.3% 1 to 2 gtts QID × 5 days, gentamicin oint ½" TID GC: ceftriaxone 1 gm IM × 1; infants 25 to 50 mg/kg IM/IV × 1 (max 125 mg)
- Contact Lens: ciprofloxacin 0.3% 1 to 2 gtts q 1 to 6 hours or 4th generation quinolone (Moxifloxacin)
- **Corneal FB:** topical anesthesia, tetanus status, removal with moistened cotton tip applicator, eye spud, sterile needle. Rust ring removal with automated burr
- **Corneal Abrasion:** topical/oral anesthesia, tetanus status, no patch. Erythromycin oint ½" QID; ciprofloxacin 0.3% 1 to 2 gtts; sulfacetamide 10% oint or gtts; ofloxacin 1 to 2 gtts q 1 to 6 hours
- Contact Lens: levofloxacin 0.5% gtts; tobramycin 0.3% 0.3% gtts; stop contact use, recheck 1 day for corneal ulcer
- **HSV:** topical/oral analgesia or cycloplegic gtt; trifluridine 1% gtts (max 9 gtts/d); acyclovir 800 mg PO five times a day × 7 to 10 days
- **Hyphema:** based on degree of hyphema. Topical/oral analgesia or cycloplegic gtts, topical/steroids, eye rest (bilateral patch), possible admit/surgery HZV: antivirals within 48 to 72 hours. Acyclovir 800 mg PO five times a day × 7 to 10 days (or valacylovir, famciclovir)
- **Iritis/Uveitis:** oral analgesia and cycloplegic gtts; consult ophth for topical steroid use such as prednisolone 1% 1 to 2 gtts q 1 hour initially
- **Orbital Cellulitis:** fever control, analgesia, baseline labs, CT orbits and/or sinuses to R/O periorbital cellulitis; admit vancomycin 20 mg/kg BID plus ampicillin/sulbactam 3 g IV or clindamycin 600 to 900 mg IV TID, or piperacillin/tazobactam 4.5 g IV QID
- **Periorbital Cellulitis:** outpt if nontoxic and F/U 1 day; admit < 1 year or if severe; warm soaks, fever control, NSAIDs. CT orbits and/or sinuses to R/O cellulitis ABX (7–10 days): amoxicillin/clavulanate 875 PO BID; cephalexin 500 mg PO QID; clindamycin 300 to 450 PO TID; ampicillin/sulbactam 3 g IV, ceftriaxone 2 g IV; add vancomycin 20 mg/kg IV BID if MRSA
- **Narrow-Angle Glaucoma:** analgesia, antiemetic, place pt supine, consult ophthalmology. Reduce IOP with acetazolamide 500 mg IV or PO plus topical beta-blocker such as timolol 1 gtt BID plus reduce inflammation with topical steroid such as prednisolone 1% 1 to 2 gtts. Possible miotic agent such as pilocarpine gtts and/or an osmotic such as Mannitol may be used
- **Retinal Detachment:** protect globe if traumatic; emergent ophthalmology referral
- **Stye (Hordeolum):** warm soaks, NSAIDs, abx for spread of infection, refer for possible drainage

EYE PAIN

DICTATION/DOCUMENTATION

- **Visual Acuity:** note whether corrective lenses used
- **Visual Fields:** FTC
- **Medical:** no periorbital soft tissue swelling, erythema, or warmth. PERRLA. EOMI intact without limitation or complaint of pain. Lids and lashes clear. Sclera and conjunctiva are clear without erythema or exudates. No tearing or drainage. No ciliary flush. No chemosis. No photophobia. Normal fundoscopic exam; no proptosis, enopthalmus, nystagmus. No APD. Note additional physical findings as indicated
- **Trauma:** no periorbital STS, ecchymosis, tenderness to palpation. No bony step-off or deformity. No palpable crepitus or subcutaneous air. PERRLA. EOMI without limitation or complaint of pain. No limitation in upward gaze. Corneal sensation normal. Sclera and conjunctiva are clear. No subconjunctival hemorrhage. No obvious FB or globe disruption. Corneas are grossly clear with no obvious hyphema.
- **Neuro:** exam as indicated

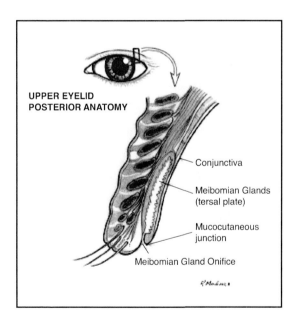

UPPER EYELID POSTERIOR ANATOMY

- Conjunctiva
- Meibomian Glands (tersal plate)
- Mucocutaneous junction
- Meibomian Gland Onifice

EYE PROCEDURE NOTE: Topical anesthetic was instilled with good anesthesia using 1 gtt of ophth anesthetic agent (e.g., proparicaine). Fluorescein stain of the R/L eye was performed without uptake of dye. No epithelial defect was noted. No FB, ulcer, or dendritic lesions. Upper lid was everted and no FB or lesions were noted. Slit lamp exam was performed. No fluorescein uptake or epithelial defect noted. Anterior chamber is clear without cell or flare. No Seidel sign. Normal saline irrigation/eye wash solution was performed and the pt tolerated the procedure well, no adverse reaction or complications. Note intraocular pressure readings.

EYE PAIN

DON'T MISS!

- Corneal ulcer
- Acute narrow angle glaucoma, >50 years
- *Pseudomonas* contact lens infection
- Intraocular FB

EARACHE

HX
- Onset, duration
- F/C, N/V/D
- Nasal discharge, congestion, sinus pain
- Cough, sputum production
- Pulling at ear, drainage, hearing loss, tinnitus, deep ear pain, blisters around ear canal or mouth
- Headache, vertigo, trouble with speech or balance
- Facial weakness or paralysis
- Local trauma, exposure to water, foreign objects, day care
- Recent altitude changes, head injury
- Poor feeding or behavior changes in children
- Immunosuppressed, DM, HIV, atopic dermatitis, psoriasis, seborrheic dermatitis
- Ramsay Hunt Syndrome (herpes zoster oticus)

PE
- **General:** alert, in no acute distress
- **VS and SaO$_2$:** fever, tachycardia, tachypnea
- **Skin:** PWD, normal texture and turgor; no lesions
- **HEENT:**
  - **Head:** NT, normal fontanel (if still open)
  - **Eyes:** PERRLA, EOMI, sclera and conjunctiva clear, drainage, periorbital STS or erythema
  - **Ears:** pre- or postauricular lymphadenopathy or erythema. Pain on movement of tragus or auricle, protrusion of auricle. Canal: erythema, edema, exudate, FB vesicular lesions of ear canal or auricle. TM: erythema, bulging, retraction, landmarks, fluid level, bullae, perforation, cerumen
  - **Nose:** rhinorrhea, flare
  - **Face:** ipsilateral facial weakness or paralysis
  - **Mouth/Throat:** MMM, posterior pharynx clear, no erythema, exudate, vesicles, petechiae, dysarthria
- **Neck:** supple, NT, FROM, no meningismus or lymphadenopathy
- **Chest:** CTA, wheezes, rhonchi, rales; retractions, O$_2$ sat
- **Abd:** soft, BSA, NT, no HSM
- **Back:** no spinal or CVAT
- **Neuro:** A&O × 4, GCS 15, no focal neuro deficits, normal behavior for age

EARACHE

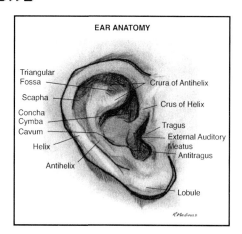

EAR ANATOMY

Triangular Fossa
Scapha
Concha
Cymba
Cavum
Helix
Antihelix
Crura of Antihelix
Crus of Helix
Tragus
External Auditory Meatus
Antitragus
Lobule

MDM/DDx

Evaluation of **ear pain (otalgia)** is directed toward determining whether the origin of pain is from the ear or referred from surrounding structures. Ear pain can be caused by **external otitis** or **otitis media, perforated TM,** or **infection of the outer ear. FB** or **cerumen impaction** can also cause ear pain. Drainage from the ear canal should prompt consideration of **ruptured TM.** Prolonged episodes of otalgia with pain deep inside or behind the ear may indicate **acute mastoiditis,** a serious infection of the temporal bone and associated with hearing loss and other complications. Consider Ramsay Hunt Syndrome in adults with acute facial neuropathy associated with ear pain or hearing loss and vesicular rash of the ear canal or area around the ear. Older adults and immunosuppressed pts should be evaluated for **malignant otitis externa,** most commonly caused by *Pseudomonas aeruginosa.* All pts with otitis media should be evaluated for **pneumonia, dehydration,** or **sepsis. Dental** or **intraoral infections** or TMJ **dysfunction** can present as acute ear pain.

MANAGEMENT

- **External Otitis:** cerumen removal if indicated, acetic acid. Possible CT/MRI if severe
  ABX: polymyxin B/neomycin/hydrocortisone 4 gtts QID; ofloxacin 0.3% sol 5 gtts BID; ciprofloxacin/hydrocortisone 3 gtts BID or dicloxacillin 500 mg QID
- **Malignant Otitis:** consider antifungals in DM, HIV, chemo
  ABX: ciprofloxacin 750 mg BID or 400 mg IV TID; ceftazidime 2 g IV TID
- **Otitis Media:** usually viral, fever control, NSAIDs, topical benzocaine/antipyrine, "wait and see" 2 to 3 days
  ABX: (7–10 days): amoxicillin 45 mg/kg BID; PCN allergic: azithromycin 10 mg/kg × 1 day then 5 mg/kg × 4 days. If ABX in last month, amoxicillin/clavulanate 45 mg/kg BID
- **Mastoiditis:** possible CT/MRI and admission
  ABX: ceftriaxone 50 mg/kg IV daily; clindaymycin 7.5 mg/kg IV QID; vancomycin 15 to 20 mg/kg BID

EARACHE

DICTATION/DOCUMENTATION

- **General:** awake and alert, not toxic appearing
- **VS and SaO$_2$** (if indicated)
- **Skin:** PWD; no evidence of atopic dermatitis, psoriasis, seborrhea
- **HEENT:**
  - **Head:** atraumatic, nontender; no scalp dermatitis
  - **Eyes:** sclera and conjunctiva clear, PERRLA, EOMI
  - **Ears:** no pre- or postauricular lymphadenopathy or erythema; canals are clear, no erythema, edema, exudates. No cerumen impaction. TMs normal without bulging or retraction. Good light reflex. No fluid level, vesicles, or bullae. No perforation
  - **Nose/Face:** no rhinorrhea, congestion; no frontal or maxillary sinus TTP
  - **Mouth/Throat:** MMM, posterior pharynx clear, no erythema or exudate
- **Neck:** supple, FROM, nontender, no lymphadenopathy, no meningismus
- **Chest:** CTA
- **Abd:** soft, BSA, NT
- **Back:** no spinal or CVAT
- **Neuro:** A&O × 4, GCS 15, no focal neuro deficits, normal behavior for age

CERUMEN REMOVAL PROCEDURE NOTE: The pt had cerumen removed from the L/R ear canal with a loop in order to visualize the TM. There were no complications.

DON'T MISS!

- Toxic appearing
- Unable to tolerate fluids; dehydration
- Meningismus
- Mastoiditis
- Malignant otitis externa
- Pneumonia

NASAL INJURY

HX
- MOI, circumstances, HA, LOC, N/V facial, nasal, neck pain
- Epistaxis, eye pain, visual changes

PE
- **General:** level of distress
- **VS and SaO$_2$** (if indicated)
- **Skin:** PWD
- **HEENT:**
  - **Head:** surface trauma, TTP, bony step-off
  - **Eyes:** periorbital ecchymosis, TTP, subconjunctival hemorrhage, EOMI, diplopia, corneas grossly clear
  - **Ears:** canals, TMs clear, ruptured TM, hemotympanum, Battle's sign
  - **Nose/Face:** surface trauma, STS, ecchymosis, deformity, epistaxis, CSF leak, internal nasal injury, septal hematoma. Midface instability, movement of superior alveolar ridge. Tenderness of zygoma, maxilla, mandible
  - **Mouth/Throat:** intraoral injury, teeth and mandible stable. Posterior pharynx clear
- **Neck:** NT, FROM. No midline point tenderness, step-off or deformity to firm palpation of posterior cervical spine. Trachea midline. Carotids equal. No masses. No JVD. FROM of the neck without limitation or pain
- **Neuro:** A&O × 4, GCS 15, CN II–XII, grossly intact, no focal neuro deficits

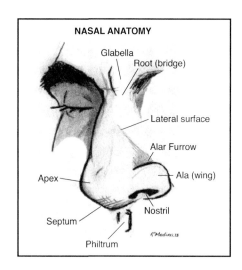

NASAL ANATOMY

Glabella

Root (bridge)

Lateral surface

Alar Furrow

Ala (wing)

Apex

Nostril

Septum

Philtrum

NASAL INJURY

MDM/DDx

An isolated nasal injury is often treated as a contusion or "**clinical nasal fracture**" without radiographic confirmation. More significant injuries include **open nasal fractures** and **associated infection** or **septal hematoma**, which can lead to permanent deformity. **Nasal trauma** can also cause significant blood loss and airway management problems. **Facial fractures** associated with nasal trauma include Le Fort fractures and orbital blow-out fracture with entrapment of EOMs. **Concurrent head injury** and/or **cervical spine injury** must always be considered in pts with nasal trauma.

MANAGEMENT

- Ice, elevate HOB, analgesia. X-rays not needed for suspected nasal FX unless open FX
- **Septal Hematoma:** Needle aspiration or I&D, ABX

DICTATION/DOCUMENTATION

- **General:** level of distress. Pt is awake and alert, no fever or tachycardia
- **VS and SaO$_2$** (if indicated)
- **Skin:** PWD
- **HEENT:**
  - **Head:** atraumatic, nontender to palpation
  - **Eyes:** sclera and conjunctiva clear, PERRLA, EOMI without limitation or pain, no periorbital step-off, ecchymosis, or deformity. No infraorbital anesthesia
  - **Ears:** TMs normal, no hemotympanum or Battle's sign
  - **Nose/Face:** no epistaxis or CSF leak, no STS, ecchymosis, or open wounds. No bony step-off or obvious deformity. No septal hematoma. No midface instability or movement of superior alveolar ridge. No bony tenderness of zygoma, maxilla, mandible
  - **Mouth/Throat:** no intraoral trauma, teeth and mandible stable. Posterior pharynx clear
- **Neck:** FROM, nontender to firm palpation of bony posterior cervical spine, no paraspinal STS or TTP
- **Neuro:** A&O × 4, GCS 15, CN II–XII, grossly intact, no focal neuro deficits

FACIAL PAIN

HX

- F/C, N/V onset, duration, quality, location, radiation
- Provoking factors trigger points
- Severe, sharp, lancinating (stabbing), electric-shock pain
- Constant or paroxysmal
- Headache: general or focal
- Postauricular headache or otalgia
- Facial weakness, droop
- Change in taste or hearing
- Blurred vision, tearing, or decreased tearing
- Dental or sinus problems
- Skin infection, HX facial HZV

PE

- **General:** level of distress
- **VS and SaO$_2$** (if indicated)
- **Skin:** PWD
- **HEENT:**
    - **Head:** scalp tenderness or trigger points
    - **Eyes:** PERRLA, tearing, redness, corneal reflex, chemosis, EOMs intact, ptosis, Bell's phenomenon (as pt closes eye, eye rolls up and in, eyelid does not close)
    - **Ears:** canals and TMs clear, pre- or postauricular lymphadenopathy
    - **Nose/Face:** nasal congestion or inflammation, frontal or maxillary sinus tenderness, STS, erythema, warmth, symmetry, facial droop, loss of nasolabial fold, facial sensation to light touch in three branches of trigeminal nerve, facial movement, trismus, TMJ, jaw click
    - **Mouth/Throat:** intraoral lesion, swelling, dental injury or infection, Wharton's duct (parotid), Stensen's duct (salivary), posterior pharynx
- **Neck:** FROM, supple, meningismus, lymphadenopathy
- **Neuro:** A&O × 4, GCS 15, CN II–XII, focal neurological deficit

MDM/DDx

Nontraumatic facial pain is often caused by **acute rhinosinusitis** or **dental problems**, which can result in **facial cellulitis**. Pts with any orbital involvement, such as **periorbital swelling, chemosis**, or **lateral gaze palsy (CN VI)**, should be evaluated for **cavernous sinus thrombosis**, a serious complication of central face, sinus, or dental infections. **Sialadenitis** or **sialolithiasis** can be caused by infection or obstruction of a salivary gland. Acute onset of complete unilateral facial paralysis indicates **Bell's palsy (CV VII)**. Also consider **Lyme disease** as cause of facial paralysis. Painful facial paralysis associated with hearing loss and periauricular vesicular rash should prompt consideration of **Ramsey Hunt syndrome**. **Trigeminal neuralgia (CN V)** should be considered in pts with unilateral, paroxysmal stabbing, or electric-shock pain. **Postherpetic neuralgia** can persist for several months after an acute HZV infection. The dull ache of **TMJ dysfunction** facial pain often radiates to the ear or head and is exacerbated by chewing and eating. Any of the spectrums of **headache syndromes** can result in radiation of pain to the face. Consider **Giant cell arteritis (temporal arteritis)** in older pts with new-onset headache, tenderness, or decreased pulsation in the temporal area.

FACIAL PAIN

MANAGEMENT

- Refer also to "Abscess/Cellulitis," or "Dental/Intraoral Pain"
- **Sinusitis:** usually viral and requires supportive care, such as fever control, analgesia, antihistamines, decongestants, possible intranasal steroids. Prolonged SXS may require: **ABX:** 10 to 14 days course: amoxicillin 1 g PO TID; TMP/SMX (DS) 1 to 2 tabs PO BID; doxycycline 100 mg PO BID; or azithromycin 500 PO mg daily × 3 days. Severe cases with facial pain, swelling, redness: amoxicillin/ clavulanate 875 mg PO BID × 10 days; levofloxacin 750 mg PO daily × 5 days. Consider fungal etiology in immunocompromised or DM pts. ENT referral for chronic sinusitis
- **Trigeminal neuralgia:** carbamazepine 100 mg PO BID; **TMJ Dysfunction:** soft diet, mouth guard, NSAIDs, muscle relaxants; **giant cell arteritis:** ESR (usually > 50), CRP, prednisone 60 to 80 mg PO/d tapered (higher dose IV if visual changes present)

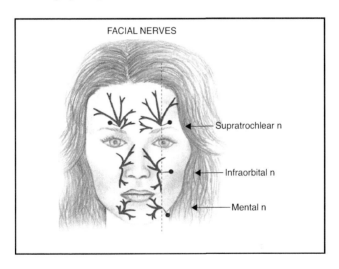

FACIAL NERVES

Supratrochlear n

Infraorbital n

Mental n

FACIAL INJURY

HX
- Time of injury, MOI: sports, assault, MVC, fall, seizure
- HA, visual problems, neck pain, LOC
- Blood or CSF from nose or ears
- HX vomiting

PE
- **General:** alert, in no distress. VS stable
- **VS and SaO$_2$**
- **Skin:** PWD
- **HEENT:**
  - **Head:** scalp contusion, tenderness, open wounds, FB, bony step-off, or deformity
  - **Eyes:** VA, PERRLA, diplopia. Sclera and conjunctiva, subconjunctival hemorrhage, hyphema, EOM intact without pain or limited upward gaze. Enophthalmos or exophthalmos. Eyelid swelling, contusion, ability to open and close lids. Ability to raise eyebrows. Periorbital ecchymosis or bony step-off. Infraorbital swelling, anesthesia, palpable subcutaneous air
  - **Ears:** canals, TMs clear, ruptured TM, hemotympanum, Battle's sign, auricular hematoma, otorrhea
  - **Nose:** deviation, TTP, STS, ecchymosis, open wound, epistaxis, CSF rhinorrhea, septal hematoma
  - **Mouth/Throat:** lip swelling or contusion. Note if lacerations cross vermillion border or through-and-through. Tongue laceration, intraoral or dental trauma, bleeding, swelling. Patent parotid duct. Posterior pharynx clear, patent airway. Malocclusion or trismus
- **Face:** asymmetry, STS, abrasions, ecchymosis, contusions, open wounds. Bony tenderness step-off, deformity of forehead, periorbital area, zygoma, flattened or mobile maxilla, TMJ, mandible. Midface instability, sensorimotor functions of face. Note clear drainage from midcheek laceration in area of parotid gland
- **Neck:** NT to firm midline palpation of posterior C-spine, FROM, spasm, mass, STS
- **Chest:** CTA
- **Abd:** soft, BSA, NT
- **Back:** spinal or CVAT
- **Extrems:** FROM, NT, good strength
- **Neuro:** A&O × 4, GCS 15, CN II–XII, no focal neurological deficit

FACIAL INJURY

MDM/DDx

Facial injuries range from soft tissue injury, such as **contusions** and **abrasions**, to complex **facial fractures**. Evaluation and management of an airway patency is of prime concern. Concurrent **intracranial** or **C-spine injury** should always be considered. **Eyelid injuries** involving the canthi, nasolacrimal duct, or lid margins require immediate specialty referral. Enophthalmos or exophthalmos may indicate **orbital FX**. Periorbital STS with ecchymosis, limited upward gaze, and infraorbital anesthesia are signs of **blowout FX** with entrapment. Barotrauma can cause **rupture of the TM** on the affected side. All **nasal injuries** should be evaluated for **septal hematoma**, which can lead to permanent deformity if left untreated. Blood or CSF leak from nose or ears is pathomnemonic for **basilar skull FX**. Le Fort maxillary FXs can occur as an isolated injury or in combination with other FX; often associated with other significant injuries. **Lip injuries** are significant if laceration through-and-through or involves the **vermillion border**. Most **tongue injuries** are minor and do not need sutures; especially small, central linear lacerations in children. Occasionally, large, gaping wounds with persistent bleeding require sutures for approximation and hemostasis. **Parotid gland injury** can be caused by soft tissue injury or lacerations of the midcheek area.

MANAGEMENT

- Airway management
- Elevate HOB, ice, analgesia
- Possible orbital/facial x-ray or CT
- Consider CSF leak
- Oral ABX if orbital FX with sinus involvement

DICTATION/DOCUMENTATION

- **General:** awake and alert, level of distress
- **VS and SaO$_2$**
- **Skin:** PWD
- **HEENT:**
  - **Head:** atraumatic, no palpable deformities. Fontanel flat (if still open)
  - **Eyes:** PERRLA, EOMI, no periorbital ecchymosis, step-off, deformity, subq air, visual acuity
  - **Ears:** TMs clear, no hemotympanum or Battle's sign, no perforation
  - **Nose/Face:** no STS, ecchymosis, abrasions or open wounds. Nose NT, no swelling, no epistaxis, or septal hematoma. Facial bones symmetric; no flattening of malar prominences. NT to palpation and stable with attempts at manipulation
  - **Mouth/Throat:** no intraoral trauma. Teeth and mandible intact. No malocclusion
- **Neck:** no point tenderness, step-off, or deformity to firm palpation of the cervical spine at the midline. No spasm or paraspinal muscle tenderness. FROM without limitation or pain
- **Neuro:** A&O × 4, GCS 15, CN II–XII grossly intact. Motor and sensory exam nonfocal. Reflexes are symmetric. Speech is clear and gait steady

⊙ TIPS

- **Halo or Ring Sign:** blood or fluid from the nose or ear may contain CSF and indicate a basilar skull FX. Place a drop of fluid on filter or tissue paper and note clear yellowish ring of CSF layer out around blood. CSF rhinorrhea or otorrhea can be confirmed by the presence of glucose by dipstick
- **Vermillion Border Lip Lacerations:** carefully place first suture to align lip margin to ensure optimal cosmetic outcome
- **Mandible FX:** increased clinical suspicion for FX if pt is unable to bite and hold a tongue depressor as it is twisted

SORE THROAT

HX
- Onset, duration
- Hoarseness, difficulty swallowing
- F/C, N/V/D
- Earache, headache, nasal discharge, congestion, sinus pain
- Cough, sputum production
- Rash, joint pain
- Genital discharge
- Sick contacts
- Tobacco use
- Oral sex

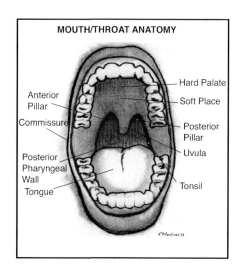

MOUTH/THROAT ANATOMY

Anterior Pillar — Hard Palate — Soft Place — Commissure — Posterior Pillar — Uvula — Posterior Pharyngeal Wall — Tongue — Tonsil

PE
- **General:** tripod position, level of distress
- **VS and SaO$_2$:** fever, tachycardia, tachypnea
- **Skin:** PWD, well-hydrated. No petechiae, purpura, scaling, blisters, peeling lesions. No rash. No lesions on palms or soles
- **HEENT:**
  - **Head:** normocephalic without evidence of trauma
  - **Eyes:** PERRLA, sclera and conjunctiva, discharge
  - **Ears:** TMs and canals
  - **Nose:** rhinorrhea, flare
  - **Mouth/Throat:** drooling, able to handle secretions, stridor or hoarseness, MMM, intraoral lesions. No strawberry tongue, no palatal petechiae. Symmetry, erythema, exudate of tonsils, and posterior pharynx. Uvula midline
- **Neck:** anterior soft tissue soft, supple. Cervical lymphadenopathy, meningismus
- **Chest:** CTA, wheezes/rhonchi
- **Heart:** RRR, no murmur, rub, or gallop, or tachycardia
- **Abd:** soft, BSA, NT, no HSM

SORE THROAT

MDM/DDx

Viral pharyngitis is a common infection of the tonsils and pharynx and often associated with a viral prodrome of conjunctivitis, runny nose, and cough. **Pharyngitis** caused by bacteria, such as group A beta-hemolytic streptococci **(GAS)**, often presents with fever, headache, and vomiting. Although there is significant overlap in clinical findings of GAS, useful indicators include fever, exudates, and tender anterior cervical lymphadenopathy with an absence of runny nose or cough. Petechiae are also often seen on the palate and posterior pharynx in both **GAS infections** and **infectious mononucleosis. Gonococcal pharyngitis** and **mononucleosis** can cause **exudative pharyngitis.** Accurate identification and treatment are important because GAS is associated with complications, such as **heart valve damage** and **acute glomerulonephritis.** Whitish plaques in the pharynx of immunocompromised pts may indicate **oral candida. Noninfectious etiologies** of sore throat also include **chronic allergies, postnasal drip,** and **GERD.** Complications of pharyngitis include peritonsillar abscess (PTA) characterized by severe sore throat, muffled "hot potato" voice, and difficulty handling secretions. **Abscess formation** causes erythema, asymmetry of the soft palate, and displacement of the uvula from the midline. Rapid onset of severe sore throat, dysphagia, and muffled voice in a pt who is drooling or in tripod position indicates **epiglottitis. Retropharyngeal abscess formation** is an uncommon deep space infection that causes sore throat associated with fever, stiff neck, drooling, and stridor. **Airway obstruction** is not common but is a potential complication in any pt with complaint of sore throat.

MANAGEMENT

- **Viral Pharyngitis:** rest, increase fluids, gargle, NSAIDs for fever and comfort
- **Bacterial Pharyngitis:** fever control, analgesia, fluids. Rapid antigen detection test or throat culture for GAS in high-risk pts. If positive, treat with ABX to prevent complication of acute rheumatic heart disease. Oral or parenteral steroids for inflammation and swelling are helpful. Most oral ABX are 10-day course: PVK 250 mg PO QID; amoxicillin 875 PO BID, cephalexin 500 mg PO QID, clindamycin 450 mg PO TID; azithromycin 500 mg PO × 1 day then 250 mg daily × 4 days; levofloxacin 500 mg PO daily × 7 days; or benzathine PCN G 1.2 mu IM × 1 dose. Peds: PVK 12.5 mg/kg PO QID; amoxicillin 25 mg/kg PO BID; amoxicillin/clavulanate 25 mg/kg PO BID; azithromycin 12 mg/kg PO daily × 5 days; or benzathine PCN G 25,000 u/kg IM × 1 dose
- **GC:** ceftriaxone 250 mg IM plus azithromycin 1 g or doxycycline 100 mg PO BID × 7 days
- **Mononucleosis:** monospot, CBC with diff (atypical lymphs), ESR. Treat with steroids
- **Peritonsillar/Retropharyngeal Abscess:** fever control, analgesia, monitor airway patency. Soft tissue lateral neck x-ray; CT neck, intraoral Ultz to identify extent. Steroids for inflammation and swelling. Amoxicillin/clavulanate 875 PO BID × 10 days; clindamycin 450 mg PO TID × 10 days; ampicillin/sulbactam 3 g IV QID; clindamycin 600 to 900 mg IV TID; piperacillin/tazobactum 4.5 g IV TID. Needle aspiration of peritonsillar abscess; ENT consult
- **Epiglottitis:** high index of suspicion for sudden deterioration and airway compromise; anticipate intubation or cricothyrotomy. Direct visualization of epiglottis by nasopharyngoscopy/laryngoscopy; ICU admit. Soft tissue lateral neck x-ray (thumb sign or vallecula sign); possible Ultz. Ceftriaxone 2 g IV QD; ampicillin/sulbactam 3 g QID; cefotaxime 2 g TID; add vancomycin 15 to 20 mg/kg IV if MRSA suspected

SORE THROAT

DICTATION/DOCUMENTATION

- **General:** level of distress; pt is awake and alert, not toxic appearing. No fever or tachycardia; no tripod position noted
- **VS and SaO$_2$:** elevated temperature, tachycardia
- **Skin:** PWD, normal texture and turgor. No lesions or rash, no petechiae. No peeling, blisters, scarlitiniform rash. No erythema of palms, soles, perineum. No desquamation of hands or feet
- **HEENT:**
  - **Head:** normocephalic, fontanel flat (if still open)
  - **Eyes:** sclera and conjunctiva clear without injection, drainage, exudate PERRLA, EOMI
  - **Ears:** no pre- or postauricular lymphadenopathy, canals, and TMs normal
  - **Nose/Face:** no rhinorrhea, congestion, no nasal flare
  - **Mouth/Throat:** no red, dry, fissured lips, strawberry tongue, MMM, intraoral lesions, tonsillopharyngeal/palatine petechiae, vesicles. Tonsillar enlargement, erythema, exudate. Uvula midline, normal size. Asymmetry of posterior pharynx. Muffled/hot potato voice. Drooling or stridor
- **Neck:** supple, FROM, NT, no lymphadenopathy, no meningismus
- **Chest:** respirations unlabored with normal TV. No dyspnea or orthopnea. CTA without wheezes, rhonchi, rales
- **Heart:** RRR, no murmur, rub, or gallop
- **Abd:** soft, BSA, NT, no HSM
- **Extrems:** moves all extremities with good strength

DON'T MISS!

- Peritonsillar abscess
- Epiglottitis
- Deep space infection
- FB

DENTAL/INTRAORAL PAIN

DENTAL TRAUMA

- **Avulsion:** complete extraction of tooth, including crown and root
- **Subluxation:** loosened tooth with blood at gingival sulcus; no displacement
- **Extrusion:** loosened tooth with partial displacement from socket
- **Intrusion:** tooth displaced into alveolar bone; associated with fracture of alveolar socket
- **Concussion:** injury to tooth that causes pain; no mobility or displacement

FRACTURE CLASSIFICATION

- **Ellis I:** involves only enamel. Teeth stable, NT
- **Ellis II:** involves enamel and dentin. TTP and precussion. Visible exposed yellow dentin
- **Ellis III:** involves enamel, dentin, and pulp. TTP with visible blood at center of tooth

DENTAL INFECTIONS

HX

- Pain, swelling, temperature sensitivity, fever, difficulty swallowing, breathing, opening mouth

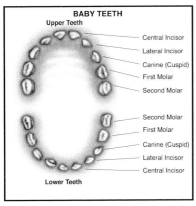

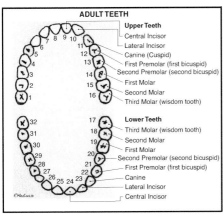

DENTAL/INTRAORAL PAIN

PE

- **General:** use default
- **VS and SaO$_2$** (if indicated)
- **Skin:** PWD
- **Facial:** swelling, neck swelling/lymphadenopathy
- **Mouth/Throat:** use default
- **Teeth:** normal, broken, or decayed teeth, gingival swelling and erythema, tender to percussion. **Periodontal:** involves tissue surrounding the teeth. **Periapical:** infection at root of tooth caused by caries. Often presents with facial swelling, fever, malaise. Requires root canal or extraction. May extend to periosteum. May see small draining fistula on gingiva of periapical abscess tooth (parulis). **Pericoronal:** tissue over impacted tooth inflamed and infected; tooth not involved
- **Avulsed Tooth:** handle tooth gently by crown; do not clean. Place in Hanks solution, milk, saline, saliva. Remove clots, replantation within 30 minutes
- **Molar Infections With Spread to Mandibular Areas:**
  - **Sublingual:** swelling of floor of mouth, possible elevation of tongue
  - **Submental:** midline induration under chin
  - **Submandibular:** tenderness and swelling of angle of jaw, trismus
- **Retropharyngeal Space:** sore throat with normal exam, pain, stiff neck, dysphagia, hot potato voice, stridor
- **Ludwig's Angina:** brawny, board-like induration of soft tissues of anterior neck rapidly causes airway compromise
- **Upper Teeth Infections:** Facial swelling at nasolabial fold may extend to infraorbital area and cause cavernous sinus thrombosis (headache, fever, periorbital swelling, chemosis/bloody chemosis, visual changes)
- **Dry Socket (Alveolar Osteitis):** Severe pain, foul odor, grayish debris at socket 4 to 5 days after extraction. Gentle cleansing, sedative dressing such as oil of cloves, analgesia
- **Gingivitis:** Inflammation of tissue of gums
- **Acute Necrotizing Ulcerative Gingivitis (ANUG):** swollen, red gums with ulcers, foul odor, easy bleeding, devitalized tissue
- **Sialolithiasis (Duct Stone):** Wharton's duct (submandibular), Stensen's duct (parotid); Sialoadenitis ductal inflammation or infection: Hydration, warm soaks, massage, sour candy. Possible ABX

MANAGEMENT

Infection often caused by polymicrobial organisms. ABX (10 days course):

- PVK 500 mg PO QID; amoxicillin/clavulanate 875 PO BID; clindamycin 300 to 450 PO TID or clindamycin 600 to 900 mg IV TID or ampicillin/sulbactam 3 g IV q 6 hours
- ABX prophylaxis indicated for Ellis II and III FX

○ TIPS

- Be wary of dental infections in pts with diabetes, chemotherapy with neutropenia
- Watch for airway compromise, sepsis, Ludwig's angina

CERVICAL INJURY

HX

- Time of injury
- MOI: flexion, extension, rotation, lateral flexion, axial loading, penetrating trauma (type of weapon)
- Circumstances: sports, assault, MVC/motorcycle (speed in MPH, seat belt use, location in vehicle, air bag deployment, extent of car damage, ejection, extrication), fall, seizure, diving. Choking or hanging. Suicide/homicide
- ALOC: gradual or sudden, brief lucid interval
- Airway obstruction, able to speak, hoarse, dysphagia, dyspnea
- Headache, visual changes, face/neck pain, seizure, N/V
- Blood/CSF leak from nose/ears
- Back/shoulder pain (cervical, thoracic, lumbosacral)
- Paresthesia, weakness, paresis, plegia
- Age > 60, blood thinners, drugs, ETOH
- Distracting injury (e.g., extremity injury)

PEDS

- Serious MVC, unrestrained, auto vs. pedestrian
- Concern for basilar skull FX, skull penetration
- Large scalp hematoma
- Fall > 3 ft or > 5 steps or > 3 × child's height
- ALOC, irritable, lethargic
- SCIWORA: neuro deficit on scene then temp resolves, then paralysis

PE

- **General:** position of pt (e.g., full spinal precautions), level of distress
- **VS and SaO$_2$:** bradycardia and hypotension indicate neurogenic shock; hypothermia due to poikilothermia (inability to regulate core temperature)
- **Skin:** warm, dry, flushed skin (neurogenic shock), pulse oxygen
- **HEENT:**
    - **Head:** scalp contusion, tenderness, open wounds, FB, bony step-off, or deformity
    - **Eyes:** PERRLA, EOMI, subconjunctival hemorrhage, petechiae, periorbital ecchymosis
    - **Ears:** Battle's sign, hemotympanum, CSF otorrhea
    - **Nose/Face:** septal hematoma, epistaxis, CSF rhinorrhea, facial petechiae, TTP, symmetry, trauma
    - **Mouth/Throat:** drooling, stridor, intraoral bleeding; teeth and mandible
- **Neck:** surface trauma, open wounds, soft tissue or muscle tenderness, trachea midline, tenderness over larynx; subcutaneous emphysema or crepitus. Bony TTP, step-off or deformity to firm palpation at posterior midline. FROM without limitation or pain, flexion, extension, lateral bending, rotation, and axial load
- **Chest:** surface trauma, symmetry, tenderness, hypoventilation, CTA, hemoptysis
- **Heart:** RRR, tachycardia or bradycardia
- **Abd:** surface trauma, BSA, tenderness, guarding, rigidity, bladder distension
- **Back:** surface trauma, spinal or CVAT
- **Neuro:** A&O × 4, GCS 15, CN II–XII, no focal neuro deficits, grip strength, reflex strength or flaccid, bulbocavernosus reflex (monitor rectal sphincter tone in response to gentle tug on urinary catheter or squeeze glans penis, + Babinski reflex (abnormal extension of toes)
- **GU:** femoral pulses; priapism (involuntary erection) indicating a high cervical cord injury, urinary retention
- **Rectal:** saddle anesthesia, anal wink, sphincter tone, fecal incontinence
- **Extrems:** FROM, NT, distal CMS intact; assess proximal and distal muscle strength and sensation and compare to other side

CERVICAL INJURY

MDM/DDx

Cervical spine injuries often are self-limiting, such as **muscle strain**, **spasm,** or **torticollis**, and do not involve upper extremity paresthesia. More serious are **ligamentous injury**, **fracture**, or **subluxation**. It is possible to have a **SCIWORA**. **Spinal cord injury** must be considered in every Pt presenting with C/O of neck pain. Emergent findings are flaccid paralysis, loss of bowel and bladder reflexes and tone, and hemodynamic instability. Overlooked spine injuries can have devastating effects and suspicion for serious injury based on mechanism of injury is essential.

MANAGEMENT

- Full spinal immobilization (rigid collar, long back board, bilateral head support, body restraints/straps)
- Ice, NSAIDs, opioids, (steroids controversial)
- Possible C-spine x-ray (three view or five view) or CT based on MOI, use NEXUS criteria, MRI for ligamentous injury
- **Note:** Cross-table lateral film alone is not adequate

X-RAYS (C-SPINE CRITERIA): Cross-table lateral view is not sufficient to clear a C-spine. Must be able to visualize all C1 to C7 and T1 vertebrae C2 vertebra. Most common injury followed by C6 and C7 injury

DICTATION/DOCUMENTATION

- **General:** use default and state position of pt (e.g., full spinal precautions), level of distress/pain. Awake and alert in no distress; no odor of ETOH
- **VS and SaO$_2$**
- **Skin:** PWD, no surface trauma
- **HEENT:**
    - **Head:** traumatic, no palpable soft tissue or bony deformities. Fontanele flat (if still open)
    - **Eyes:** PERRLA, EOMI, no subconjunctival hemorrhage, petechiae, periorbital ecchymosis
    - **Ears:** TMs clear, no hemotympanum or Battle's sign
    - **Nose/Face:** atraumatic, no asymmetry, no epistaxis or septal hematoma. Facial bones symmetric, NT to palpation and stable with attempts at manipulation
    - **Mouth/Throat:** voice clear, no pain with speaking; no drooling or stridor; no intraoral trauma, teeth and mandible are intact
- **Neck:** no surface trauma, open wounds, soft tissue, or muscle tenderness or spasm; trachea midline, NT over larynx. No subq emphysema or crepitus. No bony tenderness, step-off or deformity to firm palp at posterior midline. FROM without limitation or pain; normal flexion, extension, lateral bending, rotation, and axial load
- **Chest:** no surface trauma or asymmetry. NT without crepitus or deformity. Normal tidal volume. CTA. SaO$_2$ > 94% WNL
- **Heart:** RRR. All peripheral pulses are intact and equal
- **Abd:** nondistended without abrasions or ecchymosis. BSA. NT, guarding or rebound. No masses. Good femoral pulses
- **Back:** NT without step-off or deformity to firm palpation of the thoracic and lumbar spine. No contusions, ecchymosis, or abrasions are noted
- **GU:** normal external genitalia with no blood at the meatus (if applicable). No priapism
- **Pelvis:** NT to palpation and stable to compression
- **Rectal:** normal tone. No rectal wall tenderness or mass. Stool is brown and heme negative (if applicable)
- **Extrems:** no surface trauma. FROM. Distal motor, neurovascular supply is intact
- **Neuro:** A&O × 4, GCS 15, CN II–XII grossly intact. C/M/S intact. No focal neuro deficits

CERVICAL INJURY

C-SPINE CLEARANCE CRITERIA: Evidence-based criteria used to "clear" pt with potential cervical spine injury without radiographs
- No posterior midline cervical spine tenderness
- No evidence of intoxication is present
- Normal level of alertness
- No focal neurologic deficit is present
- No painful distracting injury
- **High Risk:** > 65 years; always consider head injury
- **Low Risk:** simple rear-end collision, able to ambulate, gradual or delayed onset of neck pain, no specific midline cervical spine tenderness, able to rotate neck 45°

Adapted from Stiell, I. G., Clement, C. M., McKnight, R. D., Brison, R., Schull, M. J., Rowe, B. H., … Wells, G. A. (2003). The Canadian c-spine rule versus the NEXUS low-risk criteria in pts with trauma. *New England Journal of Medicine, 349*(26), 2510–2518.

DON'T MISS!

- Flaccid, no reflexes, loss of anal sphincter tone, incontinence, priapism
- Hypotension, bradycardia, flushed, dry, warm skin
- Ileus, urinary retention, poikilothermia
- SCIWORA

COUGH/SOB

HX
- Onset, duration of cough, or SOB
- Cough dry, productive, nocturnal, hemoptysis
- Sputum production—color, amount, consistency
- F/C, N/V
- Chest pain, abd pain, dizziness
- Leg pain or swelling
- Fatigue, malaise
- Dyspnea, orthopnea, PND
- Postnasal drip/sinus congestion
- Post-tussive emesis
- Smoker, second-hand smoke, environmental irritants, travel, sick contacts
- Night sweats, weight loss
- HX: hospitalizations/intubation, steroids, home O_2
- HIV/TB risk factors
- IVDA or illicit drug use (e.g., cocaine)
- FB ingestion
- PE risk factors
- HX: GERD, recent surgery, AC inhibitor use, DM
- FH: cancer, AAA/TAD, first degree relative, HTN, connective tissue disease (e.g., Marfan's syndrome), MI/ACS, hyperlipidemia
- Preterm infants [(e.g., RSV) 2–9 months]

PE
- **General:** F/C, fatigue, malaise
- **VS and SaO$_2$**
- **Skin:** rash, cyanosis
- **HEENT:**
    - **Head:** normocephalic
    - **Eyes:** discharge, edema, erythema
    - **Ears:** TMs and canals clear
    - **Nose:** rhinorrhea, flare, boggy, hyperemic, sinuses TTP/erythema
    - **Mouth/Throat:** MMM, erythema, exudate, stridor
- **Neck:** supple, FROM, lymphadenopathy, meningismus, JVD
- **Chest:** retractions, accessory muscle use, TV, grunting. CTA, wheezes, rales, rhonchi, pleural friction rub, dyspnea, orthopnea, tripod. Able to speak easily in full sentences
- **Heart:** RRR, no murmur, rub, or gallop
- **Abd:** soft, NT
- **Extrems:** STS, edema, status of upper extrem circulation

COUGH/SOB

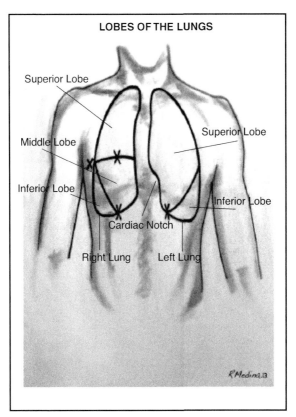

LOBES OF THE LUNGS

Superior Lobe

Superior Lobe

Middle Lobe

Inferior Lobe

Inferior Lobe

Cardiac Notch

Right Lung   Left Lung

R Medina.13

Adapted from Fine, M. J., Auble, T. E., Yealy, D. M., Hanusa, B. H., Weissfeld, L. A., Singer, D. E., ... Kapoor, W. N. (1997). A prediction rule to identify low-risk pts with community acquired pneumonia. *New England Journal of Medicine, 336,* 243–50.

MDM/DDx

Potential Dxs for cough and SOB range from benign and self-limiting problems such as **GERD, URI,** or **mild asthma** to **resp failure.** Common causes are **bronchitis** or **pneumonia** or **exacerbation** of **asthma/COPD. Cardiac-related SOB** must be considered in pts with significant medical problems. Sudden, severe chest pain/SOB with pain radiating to the abd/back may indicate **AAA/TAD. Spontaneous pneumothorax** is more common in younger adults who are thin, smokers, or have **Marfan's syndrome.** PE can present with a wide range of SXS and may be very subtle and should be included in every evaluation of chest pain/SOB (see PE). **FB aspiration** may occur in children and **aspiration pneumonia** in older adults. Children must be carefully evaluated for **resp fatigue** and **impending resp failure.**

COUGH/SOB

MANAGEMENT

- **URI:** supportive care, fever control, antihistamine if allergic
- **Asthma/COPD:** bronchodilators, steroids, ABX for PNA. CXR if F/C or suspect infiltrate. Admit if refractory to HHN, retraction, hypoxia, fatigue, repeat recent visits, HX resp failure
- **Bronchitis:** supportive care, fever control, cough suppression, bronchodilators, steroids, NSAIDs, mucolytics. Add ABX if AECB, DM, CHF, steroids, >65 years with acute cough, ABX (7–10 days): azithromycin 500 mg × 1 then 250 mg QD × 4 days; amoxicillin 875 mg BID;TMP/SMX (DS) 1 to 2 tab; amoxicillin/clavulanate 875 mg BID; levofloxacin 500 mg QD. CXR if F/C, CP, suspect infiltrate
- **Pertussis:** if cough > 2 weeks: Azithromycin 500 mg × 1 then 250 mg QD × 4 days (<6 months 10 mg/kg × 5 days); erythromycin 500 mg QID (>1 month 10 mg/kg) × 14 days; TMP/SMX (DS) 1 to 2 tabs BID × 14 days
- **Pneumonia:** based on severity and need for hospitalization: hypoxia, vomiting, septic, >65 years, unreliable
- **"Sick Pts":** O_2, IV NS bolus, CBC, BMP, lactate, blood/sputum cx, CXR
- **Outpt:** ABX choice based on many factors, such as outpt or inpatient treatment, age, CAP, AIDS, aspiration, lung disease, recent admit. ABX (7–10 days): azithromycin 500 mg PO × 1 then 250 mg PO daily × 4 days, doxycycline 100 mg PO BID, levofloxacin 500 mg PO daily, amoxicillin 500 mg PO TID, amoxicillin/clavulanate 875 mg PO BID
- **CXR:** document baseline; may defer if stable and treatment unchanged
- **AAA/thoracic aortic dissection:** CXR, Ultz, CT, angiogram, MRA

❍ TIPS

ADULT COMMUNITY ACQUIRED PNEUMONIA (CAP) RISK FACTORS

- Male > female, nursing home
- HX: cancer, CVA, CHF, liver or renal Dx
- ALOC; hypo/hyperthermia, HR > 124, RR > 30, BP < 90; SaO_2 < 90, pH < 7.35; BUN > 30; Na <130; glucose > 250; Hct < 30; pleural effusion

DON'T MISS!

- Pulmonary embolus
- Pneumothorax
- Pneumomediastinum
- FB aspiration
- Witnessed apneic episode
- Apparent life-threatening event

COUGH/SOB

DICTATION/DOCUMENTATION

- **General:** awake and alert, in no obvious resp distress
- **VS and SaO$_2$**
- **Skin:** PWD, no cyanosis or pallor
- **HEENT:**
  - **Head:** Normopcephalic
  - **Eyes:** PERRLA, sclera and conjunctiva clear
  - **Ears:** canals and TMs normal
  - **Nose:** no rhinorrhea or nasal flare
  - **Mouth/Throat:** MMM, posterior pharynx clear
- **Neck:** supple, FROM, no JVD, trachea midline
- **Chest:** no orthopnea or dyspnea. Able to speak in complete sentences, no retractions or accessory muscle use, no tripod position, infant—no grunting, stridor, or head bobbing. CTA bilaterally, no wheezes, rhonchi, rales
- **Heart:** RRR, no murmur, rub, or gallop
- **Abd:** soft, NT
- **Extrems:** no swelling, edema, tenderness

CXR INTERPRETATION NOTE: Note whether one- or two-view chest film done. No bony abnormality (i.e., no DJD, lytic lesions, rib FX). Heart is normal size, no cardiomegaly. Lungs reveal no pneumothorax, hyperinflation, infiltrate, effusion, mass, or cavitation (TB) or FB aspiration. Mediastinum not widened, no pneumomediastinum, no hilar adenopathy or tracheal deviation.

CHEST PAIN

HX

- P = **Provoking/precipitating factors:** alleviating factors
- Q = **Quality:** heavy, achy, tight (esp. in women)
- R = **Radiation/region:** migration or movement of pain (AAA/TAD)
- S = **Severity:** pain scale 1–10
- T = **Timing:** of onset, duration, time of day
- Jaw pain, hoarseness, painful swallowing, heartburn, hematemesis, melena, SOB, exertional dyspnea = risk factor, F/C, N/V, indigestion, diaphoresis, dizzy, syncope, cough, hemoptysis
- Back/flank pain, abd/epigastric pain
- Fatigue, malaise, exertional dyspnea, PND, leg pain/STS
- Recent viral illness or surgical procedures; prosthetic heart valve, pacemaker
- **FH:** AAA/TAD, first-degree relative, prior AAA/TAD, connective tissue disease (e.g., Marfan's syndrome), early sudden death
- **SH:** smoker, ETOH, IVDA, or illicit drug use
- **HX:** ACS/MI, CAD, HTN, PE, obesity, postmenopausal; previous EKG, cardiac workup, heart catheterization

Note: Women may present only with fatigue, sleeping disturbances, isolated arm pain. African American/Hispanic women are at increased risk. Chest pain begins abruptly then resolves or migrates to abd/back. Consider TAD

PE

- **General:** position of pt, level of distress
- **VS and SaO$_2$:** BP both arms
- **Skin:** pale, cool, diaphoretic, cyanosis
- **HEENT:**
  - **Head:** normocephalic
  - **Eyes:** pupils PERRLA and EOMI
  - **Ears:** TMs and canals clear
  - **Nose:** patent
  - **Mouth/Throat:** MMM
- **Neck:** FROM, trachea midline, bruits, JVD, subq emphysema
- **Chest:** NT, retractions, accessory muscle use, TV, CTA, wheezes, rales, rhonchi, pleural friction rub, dyspnea, orthopnea
- **Heart:** RRR, no murmur, rub, or gallop
- **Abd:** SNT, epigastric mass, pulsation; stool OB
- **Extrems:** STS, edema, status of upper extrem circ, femoral pulses (e.g., cardiac problems in infants)
- **Neuro:** A&O × 4, GCS 15, CN II–XII intact, no LOC and no focal neuro deficits

CHEST PAIN

MDM/DDx

Emergent causes of chest pain can lead to **sudden death** and a rapid, coordinated team approach is essential for early identification and treatment. **STEMI/ACS** should be considered in pts with left or midchest pressure, SOB, and diaphoresis. Sudden, severe chest pain radiating to the back may indicate **AAA/TAD**. **PE** can present with a wide range of SXS and may be very subtle and should be included in every evaluation of chest pain/SOB. **Spontaneous pneumothorax** is more common in younger adults who are thin, smokers, or have Marfan's syndrome. Pts with **acute cardiac tamponade** may present classic findings of dyspnea, distended neck veins, and signs of shock. **Esophageal rupture**, an uncommon cause, may be indicated by lower chest/upper abd pain, vomiting, trouble swallowing or hoarseness, crepitus, and signs of shock. More common and less serious etiologies include **pneumonia, GERD**, and **musculoskeletal pain** or **trauma.** Low-grade fever with pleuritic midchest pain that is worse with inspiration and relieved by leaning forward may indicate **pericarditis**. Chest pain with low-grade fever may also indicate **endocarditis**. Sudden SOB, altered mental status, or heart murmur in these pts should prompt a search for petechiae, splinter hemorrhages, Osler nodes, Janeway lesions, or splenomegaly. **Cocaine-related ischemia** is more common in younger people who may present with either tachycardia or bradycardia and are often hypertensive.

MANAGEMENT

- Stat EKG within 10 minutes of arrival—identify STEMI (activate STEMI team, consult/transfer), O_2, IV, EKG monitor, SaO_2 ASA (hold if dissection)
- NTG (hold NTG if hypotensive, inferior MI, erectile dysfunction meds)
- CBC, BMP, cardiac enzymes, troponin (not present in serum for 3 hours; peaks 12 hours), coags,
- Consider BNP, D-dimer, T&C
- Portable two-view CXR, serial EKGs, old EKGs if available (but do not delay treatment)
- Possible CT, ultz; other: analgesia, vasopressors, anticoagulants; cooling measures postarrest

EKG INTERPRETATION NOTE: Normal rate, normal rhythm, normal axis, and normal intervals. There was no significant ST segment or T wave changes to suggest acute ischemia or infarction.

CXR INTERPRETATION NOTE: One- or two-view chest film done. No bony abnormality (i.e., no DJD, lytic lesions, rib FX). Heart is normal size, no cardiomegaly. Lungs reveal no pneumothorax, hyperinflation, infiltrate, effusion, mass, or cavitation or FB aspiration. Mediastinum not widened, no pneumomediastinum, no hilar adenopathy or tracheal deviation.

CHEST PAIN

DICTATION/DOCUMENTATION

- **General:** awake and alert, in no obvious distress
- **VS and SaO$_2$:** BP both arms
- **Skin:** PWD, no diaphoresis, cyanosis or pallor
- **HEENT:**
  - **Head:** normocephalic
  - **Eyes:** PERRLA, sclera, and conjunctiva clear
  - **Ears:** canals and TMs normal
  - **Nose:** patent
  - **Mouth/Throat:** MMM, posterior pharynx clear
- **Neck:** supple, FROM, no JVD, trachea midline, no bruits
- **Chest:** no orthopnea or dyspnea noted; no retractions or accessory muscle use. NT, no crepitus. CTA bilaterally, no wheezes, rhonchi, rales
- **Heart:** RRR, no murmur, rub, or gallop
- **Abd:** soft, NT, BSA, no epigastric tenderness, mass, pulsation; femoral pulses
- **Back:** no CVAT
- **Extrems:** no swelling, edema, tenderness
- **Neuro:** A&O × 4, GCS 15, CN II–XII intact, no LOC and no focal neuro deficits

DON'T MISS!

- Stat EKG within 10 minutes
- Identify STEMI
- If STEMI—cath lab within ninety minutes
- Always obtain old EKG for comparison

PULMONARY EMBOLUS

HX

A thorough history regarding PE risk factors is essential because many pts have vague or atypical physical complaints ranging from fever and cough to seizures or altered mental status, or cardiovascular collapse.

- Recent surgery or trauma, CVA within last month
- Age over 60 years
- HX: DVT/PE, prior history, syncope, MI, valve dysfunction, CHF, COPD
- SLE, ulcerative colitis, or IBD
- Hypercoagulopathy, varicose veins
- Active cancer, chemotherapy, radiation therapy
- Recent prolonged bed rest, immobilization, cross-country travel
- Pregnancy, postpartum within 1 month, estrogen therapy, OC
- Obesity, smoking, IVDA
- Valve dysfunction, heart disease, afib, heart failure
- Cough, F/C, SOB, recent infection

PE

- **General:** level of distress, anxiety
- **VS and SaO$_2$:** fever, tachypnea, tachycardia
- **Skin:** PWD or pale, cool, moist
- **HEENT:**
  - **Head:** normocephalic
  - **Eyes:** pupils PERRLA and EOMI
  - **Ears:** TMs and canals clear
  - **Nose:** patent
  - **Mouth/Throat:** MMM
- **Neck:** supple, no lymphadenopathy, no meningismus, no JVD
- **Chest:** CTA or tachypnea, nonproductive cough, wheezes or rales, hypoxia, hemoptysis, sharp, pleuritic chest pain
- **Heart:** RRR, no murmur, rub, or gallop, or tachycardia
- **Abd:** BSA or TTP
- **Back:** CVAT
- **Extrems:** STS, edema; unilateral/bilateral, TTP calf/medial thigh, Homan's sign (pain with forced dorsiflexion of foot) unreliable. Possible overlying warmth, erythema, discoloration or blanched appearance; possible superficial thrombophlebitis with palpable, tender cords
- **Neuro:** A&O × 4, GCS 15, no focal neuro deficits, syncope, seizures, altered mental status

PULMONARY EMBOLUS

MDM/DDx

The diagnosis of PE is clinically challenging because presenting signs and symptoms are variable and often vague and nonspecific. Most pts with PE do not have the "classic" findings of sudden pleuritic chest pain, dyspnea, and hypoxia. As a result, this common and potentially fatal problem is often overlooked. Relevant history of risk factors for PE is the foundation for the diagnosis. Recurrent PE should always be considered in pts with a history of previous PE. The diagnosis of PE should be considered a diagnosis of exclusion when other causes have been confirmed. Problems causing similar signs and symptoms include **musculoskeletal pain, chest pain, pleurisy, pericarditis, pneumonia, hyperventilation, and others**.

MANAGEMENT

- **Low–moderate risk, young pt**: D-dimer
- **Moderate–high risk, comorbidities**: Ultz
- **High risk**: CXR, CT angio, V/Q scan (if CT not available or contraindication to contrast dye), pulmonary angiography; CBC, chem panel, ABG, troponin, BNP, EKG, possible ultz for DVT. Immediate therapeutic anticoagulation with heparin or LMWH; thrombolytics; possible surgical intervention

PULMONARY EMBOLUS RISK FACTORS:
If all criteria met in low-risk pt = < 2% risk for PE = no PE workup

- Age < 50 years
- HR < 100 BPM
- SaO_2 > 94%
- No prior PE or DVT
- No SXS DVT
- No hemoptysis
- No recent trauma/surgery
- No hormone use

Adapted from Wells, P. S., Anderson, D. R., Rodger, M., Stiell, I., Dreyer, J. F., Barnes, D., … Kovacs, M. J. (2001). Excluding pulmonary embolism at the bedside without diagnostic imaging: management of pts with suspected pulmonary embolism presenting to the emergency department by using a simple clinical model and d-dimer. *Annals of Internal Medicine, 135*(2), 98–107. Wolf, S. J., McCubbin, T. R., Feldhaus, K. M., Faragher, J. P., & Adcock, D. M. (2004). Prospective validation of Wells criteria in the evaluation of pts with suspected pulmonary embolism. *Annals of Emergency Medicine, 44*(5), 503–10.

PULMONARY EMBOLUS

DICTATION/DOCUMENTATION

- **General:** level of distress, anxiety, no acute distress
- **VS and SaO$_2$:** elevated temp, tachypnea, tachycardia
- **Skin:** PWD, no diaphoresis, cyanosis, or pallor
- **HEENT:**
    - **Head:** Normocephalic
    - **Eyes:** pupils PERRLA and EOMI
    - **Ears:** TMs and canals clear
    - **Nose:** patent
    - **Mouth/Throat:** MMM
- **Neck:** no JVD
- **Chest:** respirations unlabored, normal TV. Pt able to speak easily in complete sentences; no orthopnea or dyspnea. CTA bilaterally, no wheezing or rales. No cough or hemoptysis. No hypoxemia
- **Heart:** RRR, no murmur, rub, or gallop
- **Abd:** flat, BSA, NT to palp
- **Back:** no spinal or flank pain, no CVAT
- **Extrems:** no STS, edema, or evidence of thrombophlebitis
- **Neuro:** A&O × 4, GCS 15, no focal neuro deficits, no seizure

DON'T MISS!

- PE that masquerades as pneumonia
- PE that presents as syncope

ABDOMINAL PAIN

HX
MEDICAL
- **Onset:** sudden or gradual, pain within 14 days of onset of menstrual cycle, consider PID
- **Duration:** hours to days is more urgent, exacerbations of chronic prob
- **Localized or diffused**
- **Characteristics:** intermittent, sharp, dull, achy
- Referred pain to groin/scrotum, right or left scapula
- Pain begins abruptly then resolves or migrates to abd/back = TAD
- GI: N/V, emesis: bloody, undigested food, bilious, projectile vomiting. Constipation/diarrhea, bloody diarrhea, bowel changes, bloating, passing gas. Flank pain, urinary urgency, frequency, burning pain, hematuria
- Afib, DM, CA, hep C, GB, pancreatitis, obesity, AAA,TAD, first-degree relative, prior AAA/TAD, HTN, connective tissue disease (e.g., Marfan's syndrome) PSH–abd surgeries
- Time of last food and fluid intake
- Recent travel

PEDS
- F/C, N/V, appetite, fluid intake, wet diapers, BM
- Bilious vomiting with sudden abd pain, consider malrotation with midgut volvulus; nonbilious vomiting, consider hypertropic pyloric stenosis (2–12 weeks, up to 20 weeks)
- Abd pain in "waves," then lethargy, afebrile. Consider intussusception 3 months to 6 years; peak incidence 6 to 12 months
- Constipation/diarrhea, bowel changes, blood, pus, currant jelly stool
- Cough, chest pain, or pressure
- Sexual HX, LNMP, vaginal bleeding/discharge
- HX of same pain with new progression, STI: consider PID
- Testicular pain
- ETOH, tobacco, drugs, FH, meds

TRAUMA
- MOI (blunt vs. penetrating) assault, fall, MVC, auto/pedestrian, stabbing, GSW, missile injury

ABDOMINAL PAIN

PE
- **General:** alert, writhing, still
- **VS and SaO$_2$:** fever, tachycardia, hypotension, pulse oxygen, BP both arms if suspect thoracic aortic aneurysm
- **Skin:** PWD or pale, cool, moist; jaundice, dehydration
- **HEENT:**
    - **Head:** normocephalic
    - **Eyes:** pupils PERRLA and EOMI
    - **Ears:** TMs and canals clear
    - **Nose:** patent
    - **Mouth/Throat:** MMM
- **Neck:** supple, no lymphadenopathy, no meningismus, no JVD
- **Chest:** CTA bilaterally, no rales, rhonchi or wheezing
- **Heart:** RRR, no murmur, rub, or gallop
- **Abd:**
    - **Medical:** soft/flat/distended; BSA, guarding, rebound, rigid, tender, pulsatile masses, scars, surface trauma, hernia
    - **Trauma:** PE findings may be unreliable due to MOI. Note associated injuries, distracting pain, AMS, ETOH. Note surface trauma distention, tenderness to palpation; guarding, rebound, rigidity
      Spleen: L referred shoulder pain (Kehr's sign)
      Periumbilical ecchymosis (Cullen's sign)
      Flank ecchymosis (Grey Turner's sign)
- **Extrems:** Upper extrem circulation

LOCALIZED PAIN
- **RUQ:** GB, FHC, hepatitis, PNA, pyelonephritis, renal calc (late pregnancy with appendicitis—pt may not have RUQ not classic RLQ pain)
- **LUQ:** spleen, gastritis, PUD, PNA, pyelonephritis, renal calc
- **RLQ:** Appy, renal calc, inguinal hernia, gyn (menses, PID, cyst, ectopic, torsion, TOA), test torsion
- **LLQ:** diverticulitis, AAA, inguinal hernia, renal calc, gyn (menses, PID, cyst, ectopic, torsion, TOA), test torsion, Crohn's disease, colitis
- **Epigastric:** GERD, PUD, gastritis, pancreatitis, MI/ACS
- **Periumbilical:** pancreatitis, SBO, Appy, AGE, AAA, perforated viscous, nonspecific
- **Umbilical Pain:** poss Appy (tip of appendix may be behind umbilicus)
- **Suprapubic:** UTI, retention, prostatitis, PID (longer duration of SXS, CMT, and adnexal renderness), uterine problem
- **Chest/Back/Flank:** AAA: aorta WNL if L of midline but abnormal if palp R of midline or >3 cm

DIFFUSE PAIN
- AGE, DKA, BO, IBS, ischemia, SCD, perforated viscous, Murphy's sign, tenderness at McBurney's point
- **GU:** normal external genitalia, urinary meatus, femoral pulses, no hernia, normal testicles, cremasteric reflex
- **Rectal:** blood, pain, or mass (fecal impaction, tumor, prostate, pelvic abscess)
- **Vaginal:** CMT, os closed, no adnexal fullness or TTP
- **Back:** CVAT, ecchymosis

ABDOMINAL PAIN

MDM/DDx
In spite of many specific etiologies for abd pain, most pts are discharged home with a **nonspecific diagnosis**. Priority is on the early identification of pts with potentially life-threatening causes of abd pain. Normal temperature, hemodynamic stability, and lack of serious comorbidities are reassuring findings. Consideration of extra-abd etiologies is essential. AMI or ACS may present with upper abd pain. Sudden, severe chest pain radiating to the abd/back may indicate **AAA/TAD**. Pulmonary symptoms with tachypnea and hypoxia should prompt investigation of **PE or pneumonia**. Colicky abd pain may be caused by renal calculi or hepatobiliary causes. Metabolic problems like **DKA** can present with vague, diffuse abd pain and vomiting. Underlying inflammatory etiologies, such as **SLE or HSP**, are often associated with complaints of abd pain. **Appendicitis** may present with periumbilical or right lower abd pain but it is important that other **GU/Gyn etiologies**, such as hernia or **ovarian torsion**, are considered and ruled out. Acute abd pain in children is often due to benign and self-limiting causes such as **AGE** or **mesenteric lymphadenitis**. Diagnosis of **serious surgical problems such as appendicitis, intussusception, volvulus, strangulated hernia**, or **testicular torsion** is vital. **Intractable pain, uncontrolled vomiting, unstable vital signs**, or **altered mental status** in any pt are indications for hospital admission.

MANAGEMENT
Consider age, pain severity, hemodynamic stability, risk for serious etiology
- **High Risk:** NPO, IV, NS, analgesia, antiemetic, CBC, BMP, LFT/lipase, lactate
  Dip UA/UCG, FSBS, recheck abd, pain, fluid tolerance, poss GC/chlamydia
  CXR: infiltrate, free air, KUB/abd, EKG, RUQ Ultz; CT abd/pelvis AAA: CXR, CT, angiogram, MRA; surgical consult; abx anaerobic coverage for sepsis
- **Low Risk:** analgesia, antiemetic, dip UA/UCG, FSBS
- **Trauma:** ABCs, O_2, IV, EKG monitor, pulse ox, gastric tube, urinary catheter
  Labs: blood type screen, CBC, electrolytes and creatinine, lactate level, lipase, UA
  imaging: CXR, FAST Ultz exam (CT if stable); peritoneal lavage
- Surgical consult for exploratory laparoscopy

DICTATION/DOCUMENTATION
- **General:** level of distress, anxiety
- **VS and SaO$_2$:** elevated temp, tachypnea, tachycardia
- **Skin:** PWD, no diaphoresis, cyanosis, or pallor
- **Abd:** flat without distension. No surface trauma, scars, incisions. Bowel sounds are present in all four quadrants. NT, guarding, rigidity to palpation. NT, mass, pulsation in epigastric area. No organomegaly. Negative Murphy's sign. No periumbilical tenderness. No rebound in the lower quadrants. NT over McBurney's point. No suprapubic tenderness or distension. Good femoral pulses bilaterally. No hernia noted. No CVAT. (Include chest, GU, vaginal, rectal exam as indicated)

ABDOMINAL X-RAY INTERPRETATION NOTE: If abd plain film ordered—document condition of aorta (e.g., calcification).

ABDOMINAL PAIN

⊙ TIPS

- Pregnancy test for all females >11 and < 55 years
- Be wary of very young, old, pregnant, immunosuppressed
- Hemodynamic instability and severe abd pain = emergent pt
- Identify surgical abd and obtain early surgical consult
- Life-threatening: abd trauma, AAA/TAD, pancreatitis, bowel ischemia, perforated peptic ulcer
- A period of observation and serial re-examinations of abd pain are essential
- Take another, thorough look at "bounce-back" pts with abd pain (e.g., recurrent appendicitis)
- Negative ultz/CT does not eliminate diagnosis of appendicitis

DON'T MISS!

- Classic Triad—AAA
- Hypotension
- Abd pain
- Pulsatile abd mass

FIRST TRIMESTER BLEEDING

HX
- Onset, duration
- OB HX: gravida, para, TAB, SAB, proof of pregnancy; ABO/Rh
- Clots, cramps, passage of tissue, obvious vaginal bleed/hemorrhage/discharge, number of pads/hour
- Prenatal care, Ultz, B-hCG, previous obstetrical complications
- Abd pain, F/C, N/V, diffuse, lower quadrant, suprapubic
- Urgency, frequency, dysuria, flank or back pain

PE
- **General:** level of distress
- **VS and SaO$_2$** (if indicated)
- **Skin:** cool, pale, moist
- **Chest:** CTA or tachypnea
- **Heart:** RRR or tachycardia
- **Abd:** flat, soft, BSA. NT, no guarding, rebound, rigidity
- **Back:** no CVAT
- **Pelvic:** normal external genitalia, visible bleeding. Vaginal vault is clear, no bleeding, clots, or tissue (if speculum exam done). CMT, cervical os open or closed, uterus NT and/or normal size, adnexal tenderness or mass (if bimanual done)
- **Rectal:** blood, pain, or mass (fecal impaction, tumor, pelvic abscess)

MDM/DDx
Early bleeding occurs in 25% of all pregnancies; about 50% of women who experience bleeding will miscarry. The majority of SABs are due to a chromosomal abnormality. Other possible causes are infections, congenital anomalies, endocrine or immunologic disorders, chemical or radiation exposure. Data collection includes serial B-hCG levels, transvaginal Ultz, and baseline ABO type and Rh. In general, pregnant pts with stable VS, FHM on Ultz, no adnexal mass and no sign of acute abd can be discharged home with close F/U. **Ectopic pregnancy** should be suspected in all pts with abd pain, vaginal bleeding, B-hCG >1,500 levels, and no gestational sac. Less than half have vaginal bleeding and many have adnexal mass or tenderness. Risk factors for ectopic are IUD use, IVF or infertility, history of ectopic pregnancy, STI, PID, tubal surgery, or smoking. **Urinary tract infections** are common in pregnancy. **Other causes** of lower abd pain in pregnancy that should not be overlooked are **appendicitis, ovarian torsion,** or **tubo-ovarian abscess.**

MANAGEMENT
- Dip UA/UCG, type and Rh, B-hCG
- Possible Hgb/Hct, type and screen, cervical swabs, urine GC/chlamydia
- Transvaginal Ultz and consult as indicated. Close F/U and repeat B-hCG 48 hours
- UTI: send culture and treat (10–14 days) even if asymptomatic
- Nitrofurantoin 100 mg BID; cephalexin 500 mg QID
- N/V of pregnancy: vitamin B6 or vitamin B6 plus doxylamine as first-line pharmacotherapy

FIRST TRIMESTER BLEEDING

DICTATION/DOCUMENTATION

- **General:** awake and alert in no acute distress
- **VS and SaO$_2$:** no tachycardia or hypotension
- **Skin:** PWD or pale, cool, moist
- **Abd:** flat, BSA, NT to palpation, no guarding or rebound tenderness
- **Back:** no CVAT
- **Pelvic:** normal external genitalia, no obvious hemorrhage, no blood in vaginal vault; no discharge, no clots or tissue noted, no CMT, no adnexal masses or tenderness, cervical os closed
- **Rectal:** no blood, pain, or mass (fecal impaction, tumor, pelvic abscess)

TYPES OF MISCARRIAGES

Threatened	Bleeding < 20 weeks; closed cervix, +FHM
Complete	Complete passage of all POC
Incomplete	Passage of some, but not all POC
Inevitable	Bleeding with dilated cervix
Missed	In-utero death wth retention of embryo or fetus < 20 wks
Septic	Incomplete AB with ascending infection of adjacent structures

TERMINOLOGY

Anembryonic pregnancy	Gestational sac >18 mm without yolk sac or embryo (blighted ovum)
Ectopic pregnancy	Pregnancy anywhere outside uterus
Embryonic demise	Embryo > 5 mm without cardiac activity (missed AB)
Heterotopic pregnancy	Simultaneous intrauterine and ectopic pregnancy; risk with IVF
Subchorionic hemorrhage	Blood between the chorion and uterine wall seen on Ultz

ULTRASOUND FINDINGS

No IUP No adnexal mass B-hCG <1,500 clinically stable	Refer to gyn for repeat B-hCG in 48 hrs or admit for D&C if hemorrhage or incomplete AB
No IUP No adnexal mass, B-hCG >1,500	Consult gyn for possible ectopic pregnancy
Viable IUP	Refer to gyn for follow-up and prenatal care
Nonviable IUP	Close gyn follow-up for incomplete AB vs. ectopic or admit for hemorrhage
Gest sac < 20 mm or Fetal pole > 5 mm and no FHM	Close gyn follow-up for repeat Ultz and B-hCG Threatened AB or blighted ovum
Empty sac > 20 mm or Fetal pole > 5 mm and no FHM	Urgent gyn consultation for management of failed pregnancy

FIRST TRIMESTER BLEEDING

❯ TIPS

ULTZ GUIDELINES FOR FETAL DEVELOPMENT
- ~5 weeks: gestational sac visible
- 5.5 to 6 weeks: yolk sac visible inside gestational sac (nutrients), "double ring sign" of echogenic chorionic villi and decidua differentiates normal IUP from pseudogestational sac of ectopic
- 6.0 weeks: fetal pole visible (can measure embryo CRL; may see cardiac flutter)
- 6.5 weeks: FHM 90 to 110 bpm
- 7 to 8 weeks: FHM >140 bpm

B-hCG LEVELS
- HCG detectable 12 to 14 days after a +UCG; over 25 is positive for pregnancy; doubles every 2 to 3 days; peaks at 8 to 11 weeks; 5.5 weeks >1,500. Consider ectopic pregnancy with rising B-hCG level and no gestational sac; increased risk in pts with vaginal bleeding, abd pain, and B-hCG HCG >1,500

RhoGAM INDICATIONS
- To protect fetus from exposure to Rh negative mother during threatened abortion. RhoGAM 50 mcg IM within 72 hours of exposure to prevent maternal sensitization

DON'T MISS!
- Significant bleeding, clots, tissue
- Ectopic pregnancy
- UTI or vaginitis
- Rh- requiring RhoGAM

GENITOURINARY PAIN

HX

- **Onset:** sudden or gradual pain
- **Localized or Diffuse:** abd, flank/back, penile/scrotal, urinary meatus
- **Duration:** hours to days = more urgent, exacerbation/recurrence of chronic prob
- **Characteristics:** severity, pattern, and location of pain
- **Timing:** intermittent, sharp, dull, achy, pain with urination or intercourse
- Referred pain to abd/back/groin/scrotum
- F/C, N/V, emesis description, projectile, blood
- Urinary urgency, frequency, dysuria, hematuria
- Appetite, fluid intake, wet diapers
- Constipation/diarrhea, bowel changes, blood, pus
- Recent illness (e.g., mumps, renal calculi, or infection)
- Sexual HX (partners), LNMP, pregnant/EDC, obstetrical HX
- Vaginal bleeding or discharge
- Penetrating trauma or blunt trauma (sports injuries, assault, MVC, straddle injury)
- Aggravating or relieving factors
- **FH:** AAA/TAD first-degree relative, prior AAA/TAD, HTN, connective tissue disease (e.g., Marfan's syndrome)

PE

- **General:** alert, writhing, still, lethargic
- **VS and SaO$_2$:** fever, signs of shock
- **Skin:** PWD or pale, cool, moist; jaundice, dehydration
- **Chest:** CTA
- **Abd:** surface trauma, scars, flat or distended; bowel sounds; guarding, rebound, rigid, tender, mass
- **GU:** femoral pulses, lymphadenopathy, hernia, external genitalia, perineum, urinary meatus
    - **Male:** circumcised/uncircumcised, foreskin retraction, penis, scrotum/testes
    - **Female:** CMT, os closed, no adnexal fullness or TTP
- **Back:** spinal or CVAT
- **Rectal:** blood, pain, mass (fecal impaction, tumor, enlarged prostate, pelvic abscess)

MDM/DDx

Priority should be given to early identification of pts with emergent causes of genitourinary pain (see "Testicular Pain"). Fortunately most genitourinary complaints are related to **uncomplicated lower UTIs** and are easily treated. **Complicated UTIs** include recurrent or failed treatment, pregnancy, indwelling urinary catheter, elevated BUN/creatinine, and urinary retention. Ascending urinary tract infection **(pyelonephritis)** is a serious disease characterized by F/C/N/V, flank pain, or CVAT. Local redness and swelling of the glans penis indicates balanitis; called **balanoposthitis** when the foreskin is also infected. This local infection may lead to **phimosis**, the inability to retract the foreskin. A urological emergency in uncircumcised males is **paraphimosis**, the inability to return a retracted foreskin over the head of the penis. This is often an iatrogenic problem but also occurs after sexual activity and in nursing home pts. **Penile trauma** ranges from mild soft tissue injuries in children to urethral FBs or constrictive devices. Sudden, severe chest pain radiating to the back/flank may indicate **AAA/TAD**.

GENITOURINARY PAIN

MANAGEMENT

- **UTI:** outpatient if tolerating fluids and not toxic. TMP/SMX (DS) 1 tab PO BID × 3 days; nitrofurantoin 100 mg PO BID × 7 days; amoxicillin 500 mg PO TID × 7 days. Local *E. coli* resistance: ciprofloxacin 250 mg PO BID × 3 days; levofloxacin 250 mg daily × 3 days; nitrofurantoin 100 mg PO BID × 7 days

- **Pregnant:** may use nitrofurantoin or amoxicillin at previously suggested doses or cephalexin 500 mg PO TID × 7 days and send culture

- **Peds:** cath UA for < 2 years. For > 2 years treat 3 to 5 days unless recurrent UTI; < 2 years treat 7 to 14 days; send urine culture. TMP/SMX 5 mg/kg PO BID (> 2 months); nitrofurantoin 1.5 mg/kg PO QID, amoxicillin/clavulanic 25 mg/kg PO BID; cefixime 8 mg/kg PO daily

- **Pyelonephritis:** oral or IV fluids, fever control, analgesic, antiemetic. UA/UCG + culture. Outpt if stable, not toxic and can keep down fluids; Ceftriaxone 1 to 2 g IV followed by oral ABX. Ciprofloxacin 500 mg PO BID × 7 to 14 days; levofloxacin 750 mg PO daily × 5 days; amoxicillin 500 mg PO TID × 14 days; TMX/SMX (DS) 1 tab PO BID × 14 days; F/U 1 to 2 days. Admit for IV ABX if toxic, vomiting, refractory pain, comorbidities. Ciprofloxacin 400 mg IV BID; levofloxacin 750 mg IV QDc; ceftriaxone 1 g IV QD

- **Urinary Retention:** relieve immediately, degree and duration of retention leads to renal dysfunction. Urinary catheterization, irrigate as needed. Consider calculi, UTI, urosepsis

- **Balanitis/Balanoposthitis:** FSBS, possible culture of discharge, retract foreskin and gentle cleansing, sitz baths, screen for STI, confirm ability to void. Clotrimazole 1% BID; miconazole 2% BID; Nystatin cream BID; fluconazole 150 PO mg × 1; possible Betamethasone 0.05% cream BID to decrease inflammation

- **Peds:** if bacterial rather than fungal etiology is suspected, use Bacitracin ointment BID.

- **Paraphimosis:** emergent reduction of foreskin, ice, gentle pressure, manual reduction, surgical intervention. Urology consult

- **Penile Trauma:** analgesia, ice, elevate, UA, local wound care

DICTATION/DOCUMENTATION

- **General:** alert, writhing, still, lethargic
- **VS and SaO$_2$:** fever, signs of shock
- **Skin:** PWD or pale, cool, moist; jaundice, dehydration
- **Abd:** flat, NT, suprapubic BSA. No suprapubic tenderness or distension. No guarding or rebound
- **GU: Male:** normal external genitalia circumcised/uncircumcised male; lesions or rash. Urinary meatus clear. Foreskin retracts easily. **Female:** normal external female genitalia. No CMT, os open/closed, no adnexal fullness or TTP
- **Back:** no CVAT to percussion

GENITOURINARY PAIN

⊙ TIPS

- An inflamed appendix may cause mild pyuria, hematuria, or proteinuria
- Right adnexal tenderness may be associated with appendicitis

DON'T MISS!

- Abd/inguinal pain with little or no testicular pain may indicate emergent testicular torsion
- Isolated flank pain—always need to consider AAA/TAD

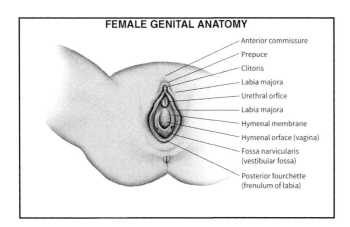

FEMALE GENITAL ANATOMY

- Anterior commissure
- Prepuce
- Clitoris
- Labia majora
- Urethral orfice
- Labia majora
- Hymenal membrane
- Hymenal orface (vagina)
- Fossa narvicularis (vestibular fossa)
- Posterior fourchette (frenulum of labia)

TESTICULAR PAIN

HX
- Age of pt
- Onset, intensity, timing
- Testicular pain, swelling
- F/C, N/V, lower abd pain, groin pain
- Dysuria, penile discharge, fatigue, myalgias, malaise
- Painful sexual activity
- Sexually active/STI
- Feels heaviness in scrotum or palp mass
- Recent parotitis
- Trauma (do not confuse mild trauma with testicular torsion)

PE
- **General:** level of distress
- **VS and SaO$_2$**
- **Skin:** PWD
- **Abd:** N/V, pain, abrasions, ecchymosis, surface trauma, or distention. Soft, no TTP, no guarding, rebound, or rigidity. No masses. Bowel sounds active in all four quadrants. No hepatosplenomegaly
- **GU:**
    - TTP, erythema, warmth, surface trauma
    - Swelling of testis and/or scrotum
    - High-riding or horizontal lie of testicle
    - Small, tender palp mass at upper pole
    - Cremasteric reflex: normal elevation of testis when inner thigh stroked F/C, N/V
    - Palp "bag of worms" (variocele)
    - Inguinal canal—reducible hernia
    - Blue dot sign: Bluish, tender nodule over upper pole of testis indicating torsion of the appendix testis
    - Penile discharge
    - Effect of elevation of testis on pain level
    - Scrotal abscess/mass/Fournier gangrene
    - Transillumination (hydrocele)
    - Soft, boggy prostate

MDM/DDx
All pts with testicular pain must be evaluated for **torsion of spermatic cord**, which is a surgical emergency. **Torsion of testicular appendage** is more common in boys < 14 years and may be associated with "blue dot sign." However, actual **testicular torsion** may be ruled out in the presence of a normal, nontender testis. **Epididymitis** and/or **orchitis and prostatitis** often result from urinary tract or sexually transmitted diseases, such as gonorrhea or chlamydia, and are often associated with systemic signs and SXS such as pain, fever and chills. Young boys with epididymitis should be referred for urological evaluation of structural abnormality. Viral illness, such as mumps, can cause orchitis. Unilateral painless scrotal swelling can be caused by **variocele** or **spermatocele** while transillumination suggests a **hydrocele**. Examination of the inguinal canal can identify the presence of a **hernia**. History of trauma raises concern for hematoma, hematocele, or rupture. **Testicular tumors** may cause painless or painful scrotal swelling. Extra testicular etiologies for referred pain include **ureteral colic** and **appendicitis**. Consider **Fournier gangrene** in any immunosuppressed pt with scrotal or perineal soft tissue necrosis.

TESTICULAR PAIN

MANAGEMENT

- **Torsion:** NSAIDs, opioids, antiemetic, elevate scrotum, maintain NPO. UA, culture, possible urine for GC/chlamydia. Confirm arterial blood flow by scrotal Doppler Ultz. Emergent urology consult, manual detorsion, surgery
- **Epididymitis/Orchitis:** NSAIDs, analgesia, elevate scrotum, ice pack. UA (pyuria/ bacteriuria), urine culture, urine GC/chlamydia, Gram stain if urethral discharge, possible CBC. Scrotal Doppler Ultz to R/O torsion
  - **Suspect STI:** doxycycline 100 mg PO BID × 10 to 14 days plus ceftriaxone 250 mg IM; or if PCN allergic, azithromycin 2 g PO × 1
  - **STI not suspected:** ciprofloxacin 500 mg PO BID × 10 to 14 days or levofloxacin 750 PO daily × 10 to 14 days. Treat sexual partners
- **Prostatitis:** UA, urine culture. High risk if urinary catheter or recent invasive procedure. Requires longer term abd
  - **Suspect STI:** doxycycline 100 mg PO BID × 14 days plus ceftriaxone 250 mg IM; ciprofloxacin 500 mg PO BID × 14 days
  - **STI not suspected:** ciprofloxacin 500 mg PO BID × 2 to 3 weeks; levofloxacin 750 mg PO daily × 2 to 3 weeks; TMP/SMX (DS) 2 tabs PO BID × 28 days

DICTATION/DOCUMENTATION

- **General:** level of distress
- **VS and SaO$_2$:** no fever, tachycardia
- **Skin:** PWD
- **Abd:** flat, BSA, NT to palp
- **Back:** no flank pain or CVAT
- **GU:** normal external genitalia of (un)circumcised male infant/toddler/child/adult. No inguinal tenderness, lesions, lymphadenopathy. No direct or indirect hernia. Foreskin retracts easily, glans penis normal. Urinary meatus clear without discharge, erythema. Penile shaft without lesions, swelling, tenderness. Scrotum without swelling, erythema, tenderness, induration, crepitus. Testis in normal position, not high riding, nontender. No localized tenderness over upper pole of testis. Transillumination, cremasteric reflex, "blue dot sign"

⊙ TIPS

- **Torsion:**
  - Cremasteric reflex is absent in torsion
  - Testicular Ultz (color) is gold standard for diagnosis
- **Hernia:**
  - **Direct:** through abd wall
  - **Indirect:** through inguinal canal
  - **Incarcerated:** reduction of hernia contents not possible
  - **Strangulated:** impaired blood flow causing ischemia and necrosis
  - Infants < 6 months at risk for intestinal obstruction due to incarcerated inguinal hernia

TESTICULAR PAIN

DON'T MISS!

- Abd/inguinal pain with little/no testicular pain may also mean testicular torsion
- Torsion is a surgical emergency (operative intervention for salvage = 6 hours)

LOW BACK PAIN

HX

- Onset, duration, intensity of pain, exact mechanism such as fall, prolonged sitting/ standing, lifting, work related
- Provoking, alleviating factors
- Prior back problems, work-up, limitations, disability, pain management
- Limitation in ROM/ambulation
- Quality and radiation of pain
- Motor or sensory changes, chronic or acute
- Pain begins abruptly then resolves or migrates to abd/back = TAD
- Bowel or bladder retention or overflow incontinence
- Metastatic disease, weight loss, cough, pain worse at night
- F/C, N/V
- Abd pain
- Urgency, frequency, dysuria, hematuria, HX of renal calculi
- Pending litigation and sent by attorney
- HX: AAA/TAD, HTN, connective tissue disease (e.g., Marfan's syndrome), MI/ACS, CAD, hyperlipidemia, obesity, DM, SH: smoker, ETOH, IVDA or illicit drug use

PE

- **General:** level of distress
- **VS and SaO$_2$** (if indicated)
- **Skin:** PWD
- **Chest:** CTA bilaterally, no rales, rhonchi or wheezing
- **Heart:** RRR, no murmur, rub, or gallop
- **Abd:** soft and NT without masses, guarding or rebound. Bowel sounds are active. No HSM
- **Back:** note gait to treatment area, symmetric, limp, antalgic, unable to bear weight. Surface trauma, soft tissue or muscle tenderness, spasm, mass
    - Point tenderness, step-off, or deformity to palpation at midline, CVAT/flank ecchymosis
    - SI notch tenderness, saddle anesthesia
    - ROM: flexion/extension/lateral bending and rotation, note if limited or causes pain
    - SLR: check for radiculopathy, positive if radiates below knee
    - Patellar reflexes: brisk, symmetric
    - Muscle strength lower extremities. Dorsiflexion/plantar flexion of ankles. Heel/toe walk
- **Extrems:** status of upper extrem circulation, femoral pulses
- **Rectal:** to assess for anal wink, rectal tone

NONORGANIC ETIOLOGY

- Pain with axial load on skull while standing
- Pain or sensory changes in nonanatomic distribution
- Flip Test: Pt seated with legs dangling, told to steady self by holding edge of bed. Quickly flip up affected leg and pt will let go and fall back, or hold pt's wrists next to hips and turn body side to side to act like testing spinal rotation. No real stress on muscles or ligaments but pt complains of pain

LOW BACK PAIN

MDM/DDx

The majority of LBP due to an **acute musculoskeletal injury or exacerbation** of a pre-existing back problem. Main focus is on potential **neurologic emergencies** or other than orthopedic etiology for complaints of pain such as **acute coronary syndrome or renal calculi**. Careful consideration of LBP "red flags" is an essential component of the examination. **Malignancy:** HX of cancer, recent weight loss, pain > 4 to 6 weeks, pain at night or at rest, ages > 50 or < 16 years. **Infection (diskitis, transverse myelitis, epidural abscess** or **hematoma**): persistent fevers, IVDA, recent bacterial infection, such as UTI or pyelonephritis, cellulitis, pneumonia. Immunosuppression from steroids, transplant, DM, HIV. **Cauda Equina Syndrome:** bilateral lower extremity pain, weakness, numbness; urinary retention followed by overflow; perineal or perianal anesthesia or poor rectal tone, progressive neurological deficits. **Herniation:** major muscle weakness (strength 3/5 or less), foot drop. Trauma: ejected from vehicle, fall from substantial height, HX osteoporosis, > 50 years, prolonged steroid use. **AAA/TAD:** atherosclerotic vascular disease, pain at night or rest, > 60 years. Sudden, severe chest/abd pain radiating to the back/flank may indicate AAA/TAD. **ACS** or **perforated viscous** may also cause acute LBP.

MANAGEMENT

- Thorough HX and PE to identify possible infectious or malignant etiology or suspected systemic disease
- Consider CBC, ESR, UA
- X-ray if MSK etiology
    - Possible plain LS spine x-rays
    - CT scan if bony pathology suspected; MRI if spinal cord, disc herniation, or soft tissue etiology suspected
- NSAIDs, TENS, opioids, alternate ice/heat for comfort
- Encourage early mobility
- STAT EKG if suspect ACS
- Ultz for AAA/TAD
- Ortho/neuro referral for pain management, physical therapy, work tolerance evaluation, possible surg intervention

DICTATION/DOCUMENTATION

- **General:** level of distress
- **VS and SaO$_2$**
- **Skin:** PWD
- **Abd:** flat, BSA, NT to palp
- **Abd:** + BS, NT to palp, no pulsatile masses, good femoral pulses
- **Back:** pt is able to ambulate to treatment area with/without assistance, or arrived by wheelchair, stretcher, or ambulance. Pt is seated/lying on the stretcher in no obvious/mild/moderate/severe distress. There is no surface trauma. Note abrasions, scars, ecchymosis, lacerations if recent trauma. No STS or muscle tenderness to palpation, no spasm or mass, no PT, step-off or deformity of the bony cervical, thoracic, or LS spine to firm palpation at the midline. No CVA tenderness to percussion, no SI notch tenderness, no saddle anesthesia. ROM—able to stand erect. Normal flexion, extension, lateral bending and rotation without limitation or complaint of pain. (Note degree of ROM.) Heel and toe walk with good strength. Dorsi-and plantar flexion with adequate/diminished strength. Straight leg raises are negative for radiculopathy. Note whether pain is increased in back, buttock, or radiation to what level of leg. Patellar reflexes equal and brisk bilaterally. Good dorsalis pedal pulses and posterior tibial pulse. Sensation to light touch is intact at the great toe web space. Normal anal wink or rectal tone

LOW BACK PAIN

LUMBAR SPINE X-RAY INTERPRETATION NOTE: Normal vertebral body and disc spaces. Normal spinal alignment, no evidence of spondylolithesis. No obvious fracture or dislocation. No lytic lesions noted. SI joints appear normal.

TESTING FOR LUMBAR NERVE ROOT COMPROMISE

Nerve root	L4	L5	S1
Pain			
Numbness			
Motor weakness	Extension of quadriceps	Dorsilflexion of great toe and foot	Plantar flexion of great toe and foot
Screening exam	Squat & rise	Heel walking	Walking on toes
Reflexes	Knee jerk diminished	None reliable	Ankle jerk diminished

LOW BACK PAIN

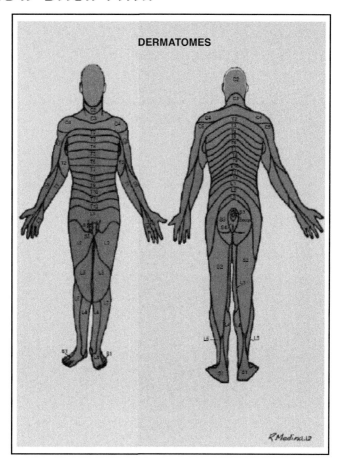

DERMATOMES

⊙ TIPS

- ▪ **Neuro Status**
- ▪ L 3 = extend quad or do deep knee bend/sensation lateral thigh
- ▪ L 4 = dorsiflexion ankle or heel walk/sensation medial thigh and ankle
- ▪ L 5 = dorsiflex great toe or toe walk/sensation lateral leg and dorsum foot
- ▪ S1 = stand on toes/sensation lateral ankle and sole of foot, ankle jerk reflex
- ▪ **Reflexes**
- ▪ 0 = no reflex
- ▪ 1 = hyporeflexia
- ▪ 2 = normal
- ▪ 3 = hyperreflexia
- ▪ 4 = clonus

SHOULDER PAIN

HX

- Onset, location, duration
- MOI
- ROM limitations, pain, F/C
- Other joints involved
- Previous shoulder problems
- Hand dominance, occupation

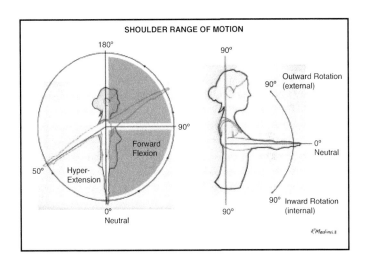

SHOULDER RANGE OF MOTION

PE

- **General:** level of distress
- **VS and SaO$_2$** (if indicated)
- **Upper Extremity—Shoulder**
  - **Note:** compare with unaffected side
  - Obvious deformity/crepitus, shoulder position, prominent humeral head, color, temp, moisture, surface trauma, ecchymosis, open wound, erythema, warmth TTP of clavicle or AC joint, acromion, scapula, humeral head
  - Bicipital groove, soft tissues, muscles—SCM, pectoral, biceps/triceps, deltoid, trapezius, rhomboid, latissimus dorsi, rotator cuff quality of pulses; distal neurovascular status
  - **ROM:** pain or limitation with active/passive movements of abduction/adduction, int/ext rotation. Sensation to light touch, sensation over deltoid–axillary nerve injury caused by shoulder dislocation or proximal humerus fracture
  - Dorsal hand numbness, weak radial nerve function
  - STS, mass
  - **Tests:** drop arm, empty can
- **Examine:** neck and chest wall for associated injury, evaluate humerus, elbow, wrist, forearm, and hand/fingers

SHOULDER PAIN

MDM/DDx

Shoulder injuries may be associated with **neurovascular compromise**. Presence of radial and ulnar pulses and capillary refill establishes integrity of peripheral circulation. Neurologic impairment is evaluated by motor function, such as resisted wrist extension (radial), resisted opposition of thumb (median), and resisted abduction of fingers (ulnar). Motor function includes abduction, rotation, internal and external rotation. Pts with **anterior shoulder dislocation (most common)** often present with arm slightly abducted, externally rotated and with loss of deltoid contour. **Posterior dislocation** should be considered in cases of seizures, lightning injuries, or other significant trauma. **Fractures** of the proximal humerus or clavicle are common findings. Other etiologies are **AC separation**, **rotator cuff tear**, **bursitis**, or **tendonitis**.

MANAGEMENT

Rest, ice, NSAIDs, opioids if needed. Obtain AP, and axial or Y view x-rays based on mechanism of injury. Urgent reduction of dislocations. Immobilize for comfort with sling or shoulder immobilizer

DICTATION/DOCUMENTATION

- **General:** level of distress
- **VS and SaO$_2$** (if indicated)
- **Shoulder:** the R/L shoulder is with/without obvious asymmetry or deformity when compared to the R/L shoulder. No surface trauma, ecchymosis, crepitus. No bony deformity or prominence of the humeral head. No erythema, warmth, swelling (nontrauma pts). NT to palpation over the clavicle, A to C joint, acromion, scapula, or humeral head. NT to palpation of the bicipital groove or soft tissues. NT to palpation of the muscles of the sternocleidomastoid, pectorals, biceps/triceps, deltoid, trapezius, rhomboid, latissimus dorsi, rotator cuff. No pain or limitation with active or passive abduction/adduction, internal/external rotation, flexion/extension. Negative "empty can" and "drop arm" test (rotator cuff). No axillary tenderness or lymphadenopathy. Normal sensation over the deltoid and ability to flex arm at elbow indicates intact axillary nerve function. Distal motor and neurovascular status is intact

X-RAY NOTE: There was no fracture, dislocation, soft tissue swelling or FB noted.

SPLINT NOTE: There was no neurovascular compromise after splint/sling application; the splint was in good alignment and the pt had good sensation and cap refill at the time of discharge.

✪ TIPS

- **AC Separation:** pain over joint, possible high-riding bony deformity palp or visible on x-ray
- **Rotator Cuff Tear:** anterolateral pain referred to deltoid, limited abduction and int rotation; drop arm test; empty can test
- **Bicipital Tendonitis:** pain over bicipital groove, by shoulder flexion, forearm supination, and/or elbow flexion

DON'T MISS!

- C-spine injury
- Peripheral nerve injury
- Occult intra-abd bleeding with referred left shoulder pain (Kehr's sign)
- Upper extremity vascular compromise due to AAA/TAD

ELBOW PAIN

HX

- F/C, onset, duration, mechanism of injury (FOOSH)
- Limitation of movement, exacerbation/radiation of pain
- Other joint involvement
- Direct trauma or distraction injury
- Hand dominance, occupation

PE

- **General:** level of distress
- **VS and SaO$_2$** (if indicated)
- **Upper Extremity—Elbow**
    - **Note:** compare with unaffected side
    - Obvious STS, surface trauma, ecchymosis, open wounds, deformity/crepitus, position (subluxed radial head-arm held semiflexed, add/pronated), focal erythema, warmth, effusion, joint irritability
    - Localized TTP over medial or lateral epicondyle, olecranon, radial head, or distal bicep. Radial/ulnar pulses ROM: flex/exten, supin/pron, pain with supination. Motor/sensory function of ulnar, median, radial nerves. Distal motor/neurovascular status
- **Examine:** shoulder, wrist and hand/fingers

MDM/DDx

Children often have minor **strains** or **subluxed radial head (nursemaid's elbow)** but occult **growth plate FX** must be considered. They are also at much higher risk for **supracondylar FXs**, which can be associated with significant swelling and **subsequent compartment syndrome**. Elbow dislocations cause severe pain and swelling. A flexed elbow with prominent olecranon suggests a **posterior dislocation**; an extended elbow with shortened upper arm and long-appearing forearm suggests an **anterior dislocation**. A **Monteggia FX** involves the proximal ulna with dislocation of the radial head. **Occult radial head FXs** are common. An elevated **anterior fat pad** or any visible posterior fat pad indicates the presence of an FX. **Clinical suspicion** of FX based on examination requires conservative management with splint and re-evaluation.

PEDS

- Children often have minor **strains** or **subluxed radial head (nursemaid's elbow)** but occult **growth plate FX** must be considered. The young are also at much higher risk for **supracondylar FXs**, which can be associated with significant swelling and **subsequent compartment syndrome**

MANAGEMENT

- Analgesia, RICE, x-ray, immobilization with sling and/or posterior splint; monitor for swelling with supracondylar FX; consult
- Subluxed radial head: no x-ray unless FX concern; manual reduction. Olecranon bursitis: compression, avoid local pressure or trauma, possible aspiration but risk of reaccumulation or introduction of infection

ELBOW PAIN

DICTATION/DOCUMENTATION

- **General:** level of distress
- **VS and SaO$_2$** (if indicated)
- **Elbow:** the R/L elbow is with/without obvious asymmetry or deformity when compared to the R/L elbow. No obvious surface trauma, ecchymosis, or soft tissue swelling. No bony tenderness to palpation of the lateral or medial epicondyle, olecranon, or radial head. No epicondylar or axillary lymphadenopathy. Normal flexion, extension, supination, pronation. Normal muscle strength. Intact motor and sensation of ulnar, median, and radial nerves

X-RAY NOTE: There was no fracture, dislocation, soft tissue swelling, or FB noted.

SPLINT NOTE: There was no neurovascular compromise after splint/sling application; the splint was in good alignment and the pt had good sensation and capillary refill at the time of discharge.

REDUCTION OF SUBLUXED RADIAL HEAD NOTE: The pt's L/R arm was grasped at the distal forearm with counter traction at the elbow. Gentle traction was applied and the forearm was **fully supinated and flexed**. There was a palpable "pop" over the radial head. After a few minutes, the pt was using the arm normally. There were no complications **OR** the pt's L/R arm was grasped at the distal forearm with counter traction at the elbow. Gentle traction was applied and the forearm was **hyperpronated**. There was a palpable "pop" over the radial head. After a few minutes, the pt was using the arm normally. There were no complications.

❏ TIPS

- **X-Ray:** good lateral film is essential; "figure 8" or hourglass sign at distal humerus. Fat pad elevation: anterior "sail sign" or any visible posterior fat pad is abnormal even if no fracture seen
- **Anterior Humeral Line:** should intersect the middle third of the capitellum on lateral view. Fractures will often displace the capitellum posteriorly
- **Radio–Capitellar Line:** line down middle of radius should bisect the capitellum in both AP and lateral view
- **Monteggia FX–Dislocation:** mid- or prox ulnar FXs—dislocated radial head
- **Note:** if FXs are intra-articular or bicondylar
- **Document Suspected Occult FX:** splint or sling for conservative management. Refer for repeat x-ray in 7 to 10 days
- **Ortho Referral:** displaced, unstable, open, or intra-articular FXs; FX > 30% radial head; FX > 3 mm or 30° displaced

DON'T MISS!

- Elevated anterior fat pad ("sail sign") or any visible posterior fat pad
- Badly displaced, intra-articular or supracondylar FX
- Peripheral nerve injury (median nerve) with supracondylar FX
- Neurovascular impairment (brachial nerve with humeral FX; ulnar nerve with olecranon FX)
- Significant STS or risk for compartment syndrome

ELBOW PAIN

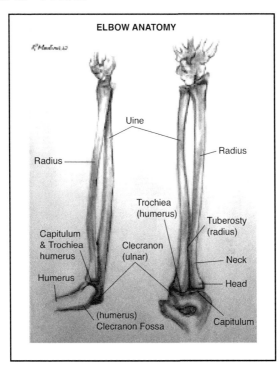

ELBOW ANATOMY

Uine

Radius

Radius

Trochiea
(humerus)

Tuberosty
(radius)

Capitulum
& Trochiea
humerus

Clecranon
(ulnar)

Neck

Humerus

Head

(humerus)
Clecranon Fossa

Capitulum

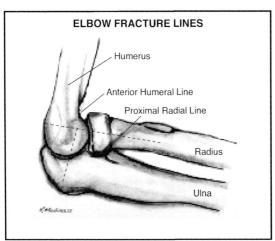

ELBOW FRACTURE LINES

Humerus

Anterior Humeral Line

Proximal Radial Line

Radius

Ulna

WRIST PAIN

HX
- MOI
- Onset, duration of pain, F/C, movement limitation, occupation/dominant hand

PE
- **General:** level of distress
- **VS and SaO$_2$** (if indicated)
- **Upper Extremity—Wrist**
  - **Note:** compare with unaffected side. Obvious STS, surface trauma, ecchymosis, open wounds, deformity/crepitus, position, erythema, warmth, focal mass
  - Focal TTP or fullness, pain over scaphoid to direct palp or axial load of thumb, pain on radial deviation
  - Radial/ulnar pulses
  - **ROM:** flex/ext, ulnar/radial deviation
  - Motor/sensory function of ulnar, median, radial nerves
  - Distal motor/neurovascular status
- **Examine:** shoulder, elbow, and hand/fingers
- **Motor/Sensory Function:** ulnar, radial, median nerves
- **Phalen's or Tinel's sign (carpal tunnel syndrome)**
- **Finkelstein test (DeQuervain's tenosynovitis)**

MDM/DDx
Most wrist fractures are **uncomplicated fractures** of the distal radius and/or ulna but can be more serious based on degree of angulation or displacement. Fracture or **ligamentous injuries** of the carpal bones are uncommon but can lead to loss of mobility and functional impairment. Hyperextension mechanism should prompt evaluation of scaphoid fracture, a common and easily missed carpal fracture. Most **scaphoid fractures** involve the narrow waist of the bone; compromised blood flow to the proximal portion of the bone can lead to avascular necrosis. Assessment of the alignment and lunate–capitate relationship is vital in the consideration of rare but serious **lunate** or **perilunate dislocations**. These injuries are most often associated with a history of extreme flexion or extension of the wrist. Soft tissue injuries, such as **sprains** or **tendonitis**, can also cause prolonged pain or instability. **Carpal tunnel** syndrome results in compressive neuropathy of the median nerve and presents with burning and numbness of the volar surface of the first 3 digits. Repetitive lifting can lead to **DeQuervain's tenosynovitis**, entrapment of the tendons of the wrist causing pain during thumb motion.

MANAGEMENT
- Ice, elevation, NSAIDs, analgesia
- Wrist brace, volar splint, ulnar gutter splint, thumb spica splint
- Conservative splinting and recheck for possible growth plate FX or scaphoid FX

WRIST PAIN

DICTATION/DOCUMENTATION

- **General:** level of distress
- **VS and SaO$_2$** (if indicated)
- **Wrist:** the R/L wrist is with/without obvious asymmetry or deformity when compared to the R/L wrist. No surface trauma, open wounds, swelling, or obvious deformity. No overlying erythema or warmth. No bony crepitus or focal area of TTP. No scaphoid fullness or tenderness to direct palpation or axial load. Normal flex/ext, ulnar/radial deviation. Motor/sensory function of ulnar, radial, median nerves intact. Ulnar and radial pulses intact
- Negative Phalen's/Tinel's sign (carpal tunnel syndrome). Negative Finkelstein test (DeQuervain's tenosynovitis)

X-RAY NOTE: There was no fracture, dislocation, soft tissue swelling or FB noted.

SPLINT NOTE: There was no neurovascular compromise after splint/sling application; the splint was in good alignment and the pt had good sensation and capillary refill at the time of discharge.

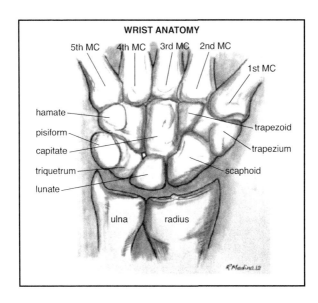

WRIST ANATOMY

5th MC   4th MC   3rd MC   2nd MC   1st MC

hamate
pisiform
capitate
triquetrum
lunate
trapezoid
trapezium
scaphoid

ulna   radius

R. Medina.12

DON'T MISS!

- Navicular/scaphoid FX—most commonly injured carpal bone, easily missed, can lead to avascular necrosis
- Lunate or perilunate dislocations

HAND PAIN

HX

- MOI: work or sports related, hyperextension/flexion, crush, forceful abduction of thumb
- Animal or human bite
- High-pressure puncture injury
- Movement limitations
- Feeling of fullness, throbbing pain, swelling of fingertip proximal lymphangitis
- Occupation, hand dominance
- Work-related injury
- Onset, duration, delayed presentation
- Pain, F/C

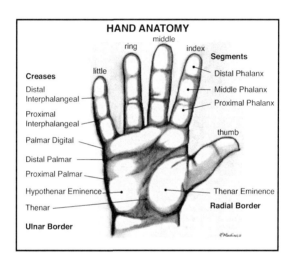

PE

- **General:** level of distress
- **VS and SaO$_2$** (if indicated)
- **Upper Extremity—Hand/Fingers**
  - **Note:** compare with unaffected side; examine open wounds under good light with bloodless field; include range of motion and against resistance and repeat under anesthesia
  - Color, temperature, ecchymosis, open wound, bleeding, erythema, warmth, exudate
  - Note local or diffuse STS or fusiform swelling of digit
  - TTP, bony step-off, crepitus, or deformity, sensation to light touch
  - Pulses and capillary refill, distal neurovascular status
  - FROM, including isolated flexor digitorum superficialis/flexor digitorum profundus (FDS/FDP) of each digit
  - Normal cascade of fingers, no malrotation (all fingers point toward scaphoid)
- **Examine:** shoulder, elbow, hand/fingers

HAND PAIN

FLEXOR TENDONS
■ FDS and FDP

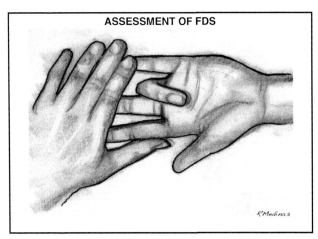

ASSESSMENT OF FDS

NOTE: Hold nonaffected digits in complete extension and evaluate strength of flexion of the PIP joint with the DIP joints in extension. It is important to eliminate use of intrinsic palmar muscles in order to isolate the flexor tendon.

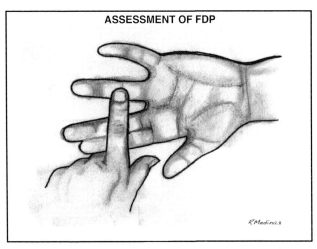

ASSESSMENT OF FDP

NOTE: Hold middle phalanx in complete extension and evaluate strength of **flexion of the distal phalax (DIP)**. Repeat for each digit.

HAND PAIN

EXTENSOR TENDONS
- **Abductor Pollicis Longus and Extensor Pollicis Brevis:** abduct thumb from other fingers
- **Extensor Carpi Radialis Longus and Extensor Carpi Radialis Brevis:** make fist and extend hand at wrist
- **Extensor Pollicis Longus:** palm down and raise thumb
- **Extensor Carpi Ulnaris:** ulnar deviation; intact extension of digits against resistance
- **Ligaments:** ulnar collateral ligament of thumb has strong opposition

NERVES
- **Ulnar Nerve:** abduct fingers against resistance, sensation on ulnar surface of little finger
- **Median Nerve:** oppose thumb and little finger, enervates palmar surface of thumb, index, middle and half of the ring finger
- **Radial Nerve:** extend wrist and fingers against resistance, sensation on dorsal web space between thumb and index finger

NAILS
- Nail avulsion, tissue avulsion, partial/complete amputation, subungual hematoma

MDM/DDx
Infections of the fingers and hand include local **paronychia, felon, cellulitis,** and **flexor tenosynovitis.** Soft tissue injuries, such as minor sprains, are common. More serious injuries involve the volar plate or lateral collateral ligament. Extensor tendon damage can result in permanent deformity such as a **mallet finger** or **Boutonniere deformity**. Strength and function of the FDS and FDP against resistance evaluates the **flexor tendons**. **Dislocated digits** should be reduced promptly and concurrent FX considered. Orthopedic consultation is needed if unable to reduce an FX, **unstable FXs** that involve > 25% of articular surface, **unstable ligamentous injury,** or potential serious **closed space infection** of a finger or hand. **Carpal tunnel syndrome** is suggested by progressive burning pain in the distribution of the median nerve.

MANAGEMENT
- **Paronychia:** warm soaks, NSAIDs. Use #10 scalpel or blunt instrument to "sweep" and elevate nail fold to promote drainage. Keep open with wick of packing gauze. Hot soaks. No ABX. Consider felon, herpetic whitlow
- **Felon:** x-ray if concern for osteomyelitis or FB. Digital block and decompress with vertical incision over volar distal phalanx, which is least likely to cause damage. Pack loosely, splint. ABX for cellulitis. If herptic whitlow is suspected I&D is contraindicated
- **Flexor Tenosynovitis:** culture discharge, including fungal, possible CBC, ESR, x-ray. Analgesia, splint in POE. ABX: cefazolin 1 to 2 g IV QID; clindamycin 600 to 900 mg IV TID. Ampicillin/sulbactam 1.5 to 3 g IV QID if immunosuppressed or bite wound
- **Mallet Finger:** analgesia, x-ray, splint DIPJ in full extension for 6 weeks
- **Boutonniere Deformity:** analgesia, x-ray, splint PIPJ in full extension for 6 weeks
- **Ulnar Collateral Ligament Injury (Gamekeeper's or Skier's Thumb):** thumb spica splint
- **Tendon Injuries:** lacerations over a tendon can sometimes be loosely approximated, the hand immobilized, prophylactic ABX given, and referred for surgical repair

HAND PAIN

DICTATION/DOCUMENTATION

- **General:** level of distress
- **VS and SaO$_2$** (if indicated)
- **Hand/Fingers:** the R/L hand is with/without obvious asymmetry or deformity when compared to the R/L hand. No swelling, erythema, atrophy, or obvious deformity. No surface trauma, open wounds, nail avulsion, tissue avulsion, partial or complete amputation, subungual hematoma, bony deformity. Normal cascade of fingers. Normal flexion and extension of fingers. FDS and FDP intact against resistance. No focal fullness, throbbing pain, swelling of fingertip. NT to palpation—describe exact joint, digit, or location. Pulses and cap refill

X-RAY NOTE: There was no fracture, dislocation, soft tissue swelling or FB noted.

SPLINT NOTE: There was no neurovascular compromise after splint application; the splint was in good alignment and the pt had good sensation and capillary refill at the time of discharge.

◻TIPS

- Consider flexor tendon involvement in any trauma to forearm, palm, or digits
- **Neuro Level:**
  - C6 = palmar surface of thumb, index, ½ of third finger
  - C7 = palmar surface third finger
  - C8 = palmar surface of fourth and fifth fingersDON'T MISS!

DON'T MISS!

- Flexor tendon injury
- Vascular injuries
- Compartment syndrome
- High-pressure penetration

HIP PAIN

HX

- Onset, duration, MOI
- Hear or feel snap or pop, pain related to activities
- Movement/ambulation limitations
- Other joint involvement
- Recent F/C, URI, night sweats, weight loss
- Back pain, numbness, tingling of lower extremities

PE

- **General:** level of distress
- **VS and SaO$_2$:** tachycardia, hypovolemic-signs of shock
- **Skin:** PWD, cool, pale, moist
- **Lower Extremity—Hip**
  - Note: compare with unaffected side, observe gait, ability to bear weight, obvious asymmetry, deformity/crepitus, ext rot/shortening, STS, surface trauma, ecchymosis, open wounds, deformity/crepitus, position, erythema, warmth, focal mass, joint irritability
  - TTP over symphysis pubis, ischial bone, iliac crest, trochanter, SI notch, buttocks, quadriceps, femoral triangle, inguinal ligament, inguinal lymphadenopathy, mass femoral pulses, distal neurovascular status
  - ROM: flex/ext, abd/adduct, int/ext rotation. ROM unlimited and without pain. Normal flexion to chest (135°), extension (30°), abduction (45°), adduction (across midline, internal/external rotation (45°)). FABER (flexion, abduction, external rotation) to distinguish hip pain from LS spine problem
  - Distal motor/neurovascular status
- **Examine:** Abd, lumbosacral spine, and lower extremity (especially knee)

MDM/DDx

MDM for hip pain includes common and benign etiologies such as **tendonitis or bursitis, muscle strain, arthritis, or degenerative lumbar disc disease**. Hip fractures must be evaluated based on the anatomic location, inherent risk factors, and need for operative intervention. More serious causes are **septic joint, AVN** (groin pain, limp, passive abduction, and int/ext rotation of leg, 25–45 years), and **SCFE** (10–16 years, M > F, obese, referred knee pain, limp, decreased ROM). Also see "Child With Limp."

MANAGEMENT

- Rest, ice, NSAIDs, opioids as needed
- **FX:** ortho consult
- **Septic Joint:** CBC, ESR, CRP, blood cultures, consult ortho for joint aspiration. X-ray, Ultz, CT/MRI for effusion. IV ABX for several weeks
- **SCFE:** analgesia, immobilize. AP and frog-lateral x-rays of the pelvis or bilateral hips. Check for position of Klein line (line from superior border of femoral neck should pass through part of femoral head and note degree of displacement). Emergent ortho consult
- **AVN:** analgesia, immobilize. AP and frog-lateral x-rays of the pelvis or bilateral hips (high incidence bilateral). Check for femoral head lucency, sclerosis, or flattening. MRI if negative x-ray but high suspicion, CT less sensitive. Urgent ortho consult

HIP PAIN

DICTATION/DOCUMENTATION

- **General:** level of distress
- **VS and SaO$_2$**
- **Hip:** pt is able to ambulate to treatment area with/without difficulty or assistance, pain, limp, antalgic gait. No surface trauma, ecchymosis. No erythema, warmth. No deformity, crepitus, or obvious asymmetry of the affected leg compared to other. No TTP over symphysis pubis, ischial bone, iliac crest, trochanter, SI notch, buttocks, quadriceps, femoral triangle, inguinal ligament. No inguinal lymphadenopathy. ROM unlimited and without pain. Normal flexion to chest (135°), extension (30°), abduction (45°), adduction (across midline, internal/external rotation [45°]). Distal motor and neurovascular status are intact

X-RAY NOTE: There was no fracture, dislocation, soft tissue swelling or FB noted.

SPLINT NOTE: There was no neurovascular compromise after splint application; the splint was in good alignment and the pt had good sensation and capillary refill at the time of discharge.

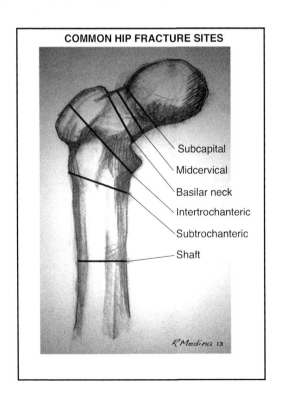

COMMON HIP FRACTURE SITES

Subcapital
Midcervical
Basilar neck
Intertrochanteric
Subtrochanteric
Shaft

R. Medina 13

HIP PAIN

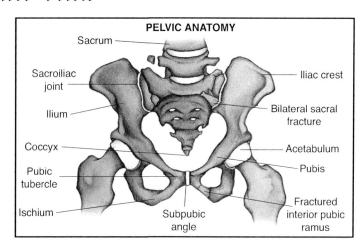

PELVIC ANATOMY

- Sacrum
- Sacroiliac joint
- Ilium
- Coccyx
- Pubic tubercle
- Ischium
- Subpubic angle
- Iliac crest
- Bilateral sacral fracture
- Acetabulum
- Pubis
- Fractured interior pubic ramus

◎ TIPS

- ▪ If unable to bear weight, consider CT/MRI of hip for occult FX
- ▪ If unable to bear weight—crutches, then recheck 1 to 2 days
- ▪ Lower extremity paresis—consider TAD

DON'T MISS!

- Intra-abd or pelvic etiology
- Septic joint

KNEE PAIN

HX
- Onset, duration, redness, pain, F/C, STS immediate/gradual, ability to bear weight
- MOI: direct trauma, foot planted/knee twisted
- Locking: unable to move passively, 45° flexed (meniscus or cruciate injury); clicking, crepitus or feeling of giving way (ACL injury)
- HX patellar or knee joint dislocation/reduction

PE
- **General:** level of distress
- **VS and SaO$_2$** (if indicated)
- **Lower Extremity: Knee**
  - **Note:** compare with unaffected side, observe gait, ability to bear weight
  - Exam often difficult due to pain and swelling. Perform knee exam with pt supine, visualize both legs from the groin to toes and compare
  - Obvious asymmetry, deformity/crepitus, patella location, STS/effusion, surface trauma, ecchymosis, open wounds, position, erythema, warmth, joint irritability TTP over patella, lat/med joint line prox fibula, popliteal pulse/fullness. ROM: flex/ext, able to do deep knee bend with symmetry (130°), fully extend knee, internal and external rotation (10°)
  - Laxity with valgus or varus stress. Distal motor/neurovascular status
  - **Effusion:** < 6 hours with cruciate lig, meniscus, FX. Slower onset and recurrent effusion more likely with meniscus injury. Patella ballottement
  - **Tibial Sag:** flex 90° and see if tibia sags posteriorly
  - **Lachman/Drawer maneuver**
  - **McMurray/Apley compression test**
- **Examine:** back, hip, ankle, and foot

MDM/DDx
Focus is on differentiating between intra-articular and extra-articular causes of knee pain. **Contusions** or **sprains** are often self-limiting. External **ligamentous injuries** are common and cause pain over lateral ligament and possible laxity of LCL or MCL. **Patellar dislocation** usually occurs laterally and must be distinguished from a **joint dislocation**, which is an orthopedic emergency. **Patellar** or **tibial plateau** fractures may require surgical intervention. Consider ruptured **Baker's cyst** or **DVT** in cases of posterior knee pain. Internal derangement injuries usually result in an effusion. **Meniscus tear** usually presents with JLT, pain with weight bearing, + McMurray test, locking, or knee giving way. ACL injury is associated with immediate severe pain, "popping" sensation, instability, + Lachman/ Drawer tests, unable to ambulate. **PCL tear** is an uncommon injury that results from fall on flexed knee or direct trauma to front of knee. Other causes of knee pain to consider include **prepatellar bursitis** (TTP over patella, swelling and redness over infrapatellar area, and inability to flex or put pressure on knee), **Legg–Calve–Perthes DX** (acute onset of limp, limited hip motion, knee pain; 4–14 years old), **Osgood–Schlatter disease** (pain and STS at site of infrapatellar tendon insertion into tibial tubercle, pain with resisted extension; 9–16 years old, M > F), **septic joint**, **gout**, or **tumor**. In cases of referred pain think of SCFE. Also see "Child With Limp."

KNEE PAIN

MANAGEMENT

- NSAIDs, analgesia, ice, immobilize with Ace wrap, knee immobilizer, or plaster long-leg splint as indicated
- **Patellar dislocation:** manual reduction for simple horizontal dislocation (lateral most common). Place pt supine, extend knee with gentle, anteromedial pressure over lateral patella to lift patella over femoral condyle. Knee immobilizer, crutches
- **Knee dislocation:** assess for vascular injury and immediate reduction, emergent ortho and/or vascular consult
- **Tibial plateau FX:** NSAIDs, analgesia, ice, immobilize, x-ray. Knee immobilizer, crutches with nonweight bearing if FX is nondisplaced or only minimally (4–10 mm) displaced. Surgery needed if open, significantly displaced, or depressed. Consider compartment syndrome

DICTATION/DOCUMENTATION

- **General:** level of distress
- **VS and SaO$_2$**
- **Knee:** pt is able to bear weight and ambulate without pain. No surface trauma, STS, or obvious effusion. No overlying erythema or warmth (medical complaints). The R/L knee is with/without obvious asymmetry or deformity when compared to the R/L knee. Pt is able to do deep knee bend with symmetry (130°), fully extend knee, internal and external rotation (10°). NT to palpation of the patella, no effusion or ballottement. NT over the infrapatellar tendon (bursitis or Osgood–Schlatter's). NT over the medial or lateral joint line, or the medial or lateral tibial plateaus. NT over the proximal fibular head. NT, fullness, or mass of the popliteal fossa. No quadriceps tenderness. No laxity of the ACL, PCL, MCL, or LCL. May note no collateral ligament laxity to valgus or varus stress. Negative Lachman/Drawer sign. Negative McMurray. Negative Apley compression and/or distraction. Distal motor and neurovascular status intact

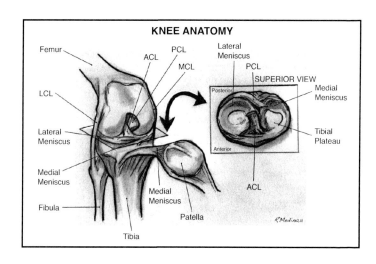

KNEE ANATOMY

Femur, ACL, PCL, MCL, Lateral Meniscus, PCL, SUPERIOR VIEW, Posterior, Medial Meniscus, LCL, Lateral Meniscus, Anterior, Tibial Plateau, Medial Meniscus, Medial Meniscus, ACL, Fibula, Patella, Tibia

R.Medina.II

KNEE PAIN

JOINT ASPIRATION PROCEDURE NOTE: The pt was placed sitting/supine position with knee supported and slightly flexed. The skin prepped with povidone–iodine solution and cleansed with NS. The site was anesthetized with 1% lidocaine ( ) mL with good anesthesia. The lateral/medial joint space was entered using an 18- or 20-gauge needle. A slight "give" was appreciated as the needle entered the joint capsule; ( ) mL fluid (clear, cloudy, bloody, fat globules) was aspirated. The needle was removed and a dry sterile antibiotic dressing was placed over the puncture site and a compression dressing (e.g., Ace wrap) was applied. Joint fluid was sent for CBC with diff, glucose, protein, crystals, and C&S. The pt tolerated the procedure well without complication.

X-RAY NOTE: There was no fracture, no effusion, dislocation, soft tissue swelling or FB noted.

SPLINT NOTE: There was no neurovascular compromise after splint/immobilizer application; the splint/immobilizer was in good alignment and the pt had good sensation and capillary refill at the time of discharge.

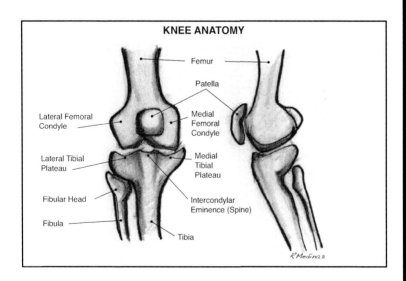

KNEE ANATOMY

Femur

Patella

Lateral Femoral Condyle

Medial Femoral Condyle

Lateral Tibial Plateau

Medial Tibial Plateau

Fibular Head

Intercondylar Eminence (Spine)

Fibula

Tibia

R Medina II

KNEE PAIN

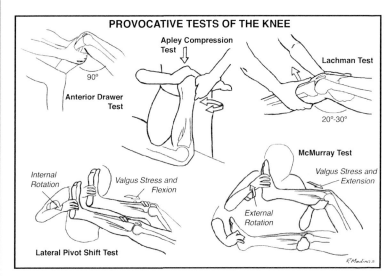

PROVOCATIVE TESTS OF THE KNEE

Apley Compression Test

Lachman Test

Anterior Drawer Test

90°

20°-30°

McMurray Test

Internal Rotation

Valgus Stress and Flexion

Valgus Stress and Extension

External Rotation

Lateral Pivot Shift Test

R.Medina.il

○ TIP

- If unable to bear weight—knee immobilizer, crutches, recheck 1 to 2 days

KNEE X-RAY ORDERING CRITERIA:
- Age 55 or older
- No TTP of knee other than patella
- PT of fibular head
- Inability to flex knee to 90°
- Inability to bear weight (four steps—unable to transfer weight twice onto each lower limb regardless of limping) both immediately and in ED

DON'T MISS!
- Subtle FXs of tibial plateau, fibular head, small avulsion FX of proximal lateral tibia
- Widened joint space—unstable ligamentous injury
- If joint dislocation—delayed SXS of vascular injury
- Compartment syndrome
- Quadriceps rupture—be sure pt can extend and resist
- Look for other cause of knee pain (hip/back especially in pediatric pts)
- Tumors—chronic pain often worse at night

Adapted from Stiell, I. G.,Wells, G. A., & Hoag, R. H. (1997). Implementation of the Ottawa Knee Rule for the use of radiography in acute knee injuries. *Journal of the American Medical Association, 278*(23), 2075–2079.

LEG ANATOMY

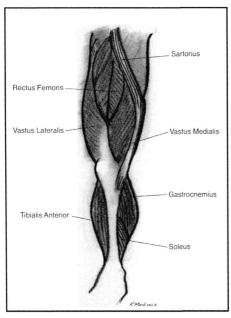

Sartorius

Rectus Femoris

Vastus Lateralis

Vastus Medialis

Gastrocnemius

Tibialis Anterior

Soleus

R. Medina. II

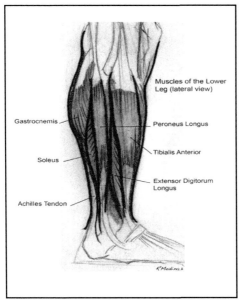

Muscles of the Lower Leg (lateral view)

Gastrocnemis

Peroneus Longus

Tibialis Anterior

Soleus

Extensor Digitorum Longus

Achilles Tendon

R. Medina. II

DEEP VEIN THROMBOSIS

DVT RISK FACTORS:
- Mild to severe leg pain and/or STS of calf, medial thigh, upper extrems
- Immobilization > 3 days, recent prolonged travel, hospitalization
- Surgery within past 4 weeks
- Recent plaster cast of lower extremity
- Active cancer
- Swelling of entire leg, may be mild to severe: pitting edema in affected leg
- Calf swelling > 3 cm when compared to unaffected leg
- Superficial nonvaricose veins with palpable, tender cords

Adapted from Wells, P. S., Owen, C., Doucette, S., Fergusson, D., & Tran, H. (2006). Does this patient have deep vein thrombosis? *Journal of the American Medical Association, 295*(2),199–207. Scarvelis, D., & Wells, P. S. (2006). Diagnosis and treatment of deep vein thrombosis. *Canadian Medical Association Journal, 175*(9), 1087–1092. Wells, P. S., Anderson, D. R., Rodger, M., Forgie, M., Kearon, C., Dreyer, J., … Kovacs, M. J. (2003). Evaluation of D-dimer in the diagnosis of suspected deep-vein thrombosis. *New England Journal of Medicine, 349*(13), 1227–1235.

HX
- CA, CVA, MI, CHF, SLE, ulcerative colitis
- Older age, obesity, varicose veins
- Smoking, estrogen therapy/OC
- Hypercoagulopathy disorders, previous DVT
- Pregnancy and immediate postpartum
- FH: DVT in first-degree relatives < 50 yrs old

PE
- **General:** level of distress
- **VS and SaO$_2$**
- **Skin:** PWD
- **Extrems:** TTP calf or medial thigh—may be absent to severe; possible overlying warmth, erythema or discoloration or blanching of skin, gangrene, poor pulses, signs of compartment syndrome, Homan's sign (including pain with forced dorsiflexion of foot)

MDM/DDx
DVT caused by clot formation in the deep veins of an extremity can cause nonspecific pain and swelling or dislodge and travel to the lungs leading to a life-threatening **pulmonary embolus**. Similar signs and symptoms can be caused **by superficial thrombophlebitis** or **varicose veins**. Soft tissue etiologies, such as local **hematoma** or **muscle injury**, should be considered. Erythema and swelling may also indicate **cellulitis**. Other systemic causes of edema include **hepatic** or **renal failure**. Phlegmasiais cerulean is a life-threatening condition that leads to extreme limb ischemia due to DVT. Consider in pts with severe leg pain and swelling, cyanosis, gangrene, compartment syndrome and signs of shock. Phlegmasia alba dolens, or "milk leg," causes a whitish discoloration—if extensive DVT leads to impaired arterial flow. Consider in women in late pregnancy or postpartum

MANAGEMENT
- Analgesia, Ultz, anticoagulants, thrombolytics (see PE list)

DEEP VEIN THROMBOSIS

DICTATION/DOCUMENTATION

- **General:** alert and in acute distress
- **VS and SaO$_2$**
- **Skin:** PWD, no cyanosis or pallor
- **Extrems:** R/L extremity with/without deformity or asymmetry when compared to the R/L. No STS or edema. No overlying erythema, warmth, discoloration. No lesions or break in skin integrity. Diameter of calves is _____ cm. Soft tissues of posterior lower leg are soft, supple, NT and no palpable cords or evidence of thrombophlebitis. No evidence of gangrene or compartment syndrome. Medial thigh is without STS or TTP. Negative Homan's sign. Possible superficial thrombophlebitis with palpable, tender cords. No proximal lymphangitis or lymphadenopathy

ANKLE PAIN

HX
- Onset, duration, pain, fever/chills
- MOI—inversion "rolled," eversion, direct trauma, step from height
- Movement/ambulation, limitations/associated injuries
- Previous ankle injury/surgery
- Recent quinolone use—tendon rupture or worsening myasthenia

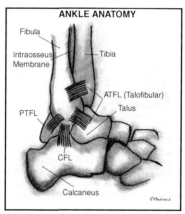

ANKLE ANATOMY

Fibula
Intraosseus Membrane
Tibia
ATFL (Talofibular)
PTFL
Talus
CFL
Calcaneus

Adapted from Stiell, I. G., Greenberg, G. H., McKnight, R. D., Nair, R. C., McDowell, I., Reardon, M., ... Maloney, J. (1993). Decision rules for the use of radiography in acute ankle injuries. Refinement and prospective validation. *Journal of the American Medical Association*, *269*(9), 1127–1132.

PE
- **General:** level of distress
- **VS and SaO$_2$** (if indicated)
- **Lower Extremity—Ankle**
  - **Note:** compare with unaffected side; observe gait, ability to bear weight. Obvious asymmetry, deformity/crepitus, STS/effusion, surface trauma, ecchymosis, open wounds, erythema, warmth, dorsalis pedis/posterior tibial pulses; distal neurovascular status
  - ROM: flexion/extension, inversion/eversion
  - TTP or deformity over anterior ankle, med/lat malleolus, navicular, proximal fifth metatarsal, calcaneous, Achilles tendon, midfoot/toes TTP, STS, ecchymosis over deltoid lig, ATFL, PTFL, CFL.
  - Thompson test—plantar flexion
  - Squeeze test—pain along midshaft of fibula when compressed with tibia (high ankle sprain of syndesmosis).
  - Talar tilt with valgus/varus stress.
  - Anterior drawer test
  - Peroneal nerve: eversion/plantar flexion
- **Note Knee Pain:** STS, effusion, pain or deformity over proximal fibula (Maisonneuve FX: proximal fibular FX with medial malleolar injury)
- **Foot and Toes:** check proximal fifth metatarsal
- **Examine Knee and Foot:** evaluate other knee, ankle, and foot/toes

ANKLE PAIN

ANKLE/FOOT X-RAY ORDERING CRITERIA:

- **Ankle X-Ray**
    - PT at posterior edge or tip of lateral malleolus
    - Age 55 or older
    - PT at posterior edge or tip of medial malleolus
- **Foot X-Ray**
    - Should be ordered if there is any pain in the midfoot zone and any of the following: PT at base of fifth metatarsal, PT at navicular
    - Age 55 or older
    - Inability to bear weight both immediately and in the ED

MDM/DDx

Ankle injuries most often involve **sprains** caused by an inversion or twisting mechanism that causes pain, ecchymosis, and STS over the ATFL or CFL. Consider **Achilles tendon rupture**, which can present as an ankle sprain. Involvement of the deltoid or medial ligaments should prompt concern for a **Maisonneuve FX** of proximal fibula. **Severe sprains** caused by complete rupture of the ligament cause immediate marked swelling, ecchymosis, and inability to bear weight and can lead to chronic instability. Point tenderness, deformity, or crepitus over the posterior edge of the medial or lateral malleolus, base of fifth metatarsal or midfoot suggests **FX**. A **distal fibula avulsion FX** is a stable injury. **Bi- or trimalleolar FXs** and Maisonneuve FX are unstable injuries requiring urgent orthopedic referral as do intra-articular and open FXs. Forced dorsiflexion and inversion injuries may cause an FX of the talus. **FX dislocations** of the ankle are rare and are associated with ruptured ligaments. These severe injuries are at high risk for neurovascular compromise if not reduced immediately.

MANAGEMENT

- Ice, elevation, NSAIDs, analgesia
- Air splint, brace, taping. Equine splint for Achilles tendon injury. Splint, crutches, NWB for severe sprain, or FX
- Gentle ROM, bear weight as tolerated
- Orthopedic consult for unstable FX: disruption of mortise, FX/dislocation, bi- or trimalleolar FX

DICTATION/DOCUMENTATION

- **General:** level of distress
- **VS and SaO$_2$**
- **Ankle:** pt is able to bear weight and ambulate without pain. The R/L ankle is with/ without obvious asymmetry or deformity when compared to the R/L ankle. Pt can flex/ext, invert/evert. No obvious surface trauma, ecchymosis, or STS. No bony TTP over the medial or lateral malleolus. Anterior talofibular ligament, posterior talofibular ligament (PTFL), calcaneofibular ligament (CFL) NT and without swelling. (May also refer to generally as medial/deltoid or lateral ligaments.) NT or deformity of the midfoot or over the proximal fifth metatarsal; good dorsalis pedis and posterior tibial pulses and sensation to light touch normal. Talar tilt test is negative for ligament laxity to valgus or varus stress. Negative anterior drawer. Peroneal nerve is intact with strong eversion and plantar flexion

ANKLE PAIN

X-RAY NOTE: There was no fracture, dislocation, soft tissue swelling, or FB noted.

SPLINT NOTE: There was no neurovascular compromise after splint application; the splint was in good alignment and the pt had good sensation and capillary refill at the time of discharge.

○ TIP
- Include knee exam with attention to tenderness over proximal fibula. Include foot/toes exam. If unable to bear weight—crutches, recheck 1 to 2 days

DON'T MISS!
- Peroneal nerve injury is an occult injury
- Achilles tendon rupture
- Check for proximal fifth metatarsal or proximal fibular fracture

FOOT PAIN

HX

- Onset, duration
- MOI, movement, ability to bear weight, ankle or knee pain or associated injuries, soft tissue infection, HX gout

PE

- **General:** level of distress
- **VS and SaO$_2$** (if indicated)
- **Lower Extremity—Foot/Toes**
  - **Note:** Compare with unaffected side; observe gait, ability to bear weight
  - Obvious asymmetry, deformity/crepitus, STS, surface trauma, ecchymosis, open wounds, erythema, warmth, dorsalis pedis/posterior tibial pulses, rash/lesions, open wound, or ulcer
  - Extensive STS resulting from crush injury—consider compartment syndrome STS, erythema, exudate, hypertrophy of nail or margins, subungual hematoma. Presence of tophi (gout)
  - Distal neurovascular status
  - TTP of talus, calcaneous, metatarsals 1 to 5, each MTPJ and IP joint, plantar/dorsal surface
  - ROM: Plantar/dorsiflexion, inversion/eversion
- **Examine:** hip, knee, and ankle

FOOT X-RAY CRITERIA: A foot x-ray should be ordered if there is any pain in the midfoot zone and any of the following: PTs at base of fifth metatarsal, PT at navicular

MDM/DDx

Injuries with neurovascular deficit, open **fractures, severe crush injury** or concern for **compartment syndrome** are orthopedic emergencies. Overuse, direct, or indirect trauma to the foot can result in soft tissue injuries, such as **contusions, sprains, tendonitis**, including plantar fasciitis or bone spurs. Undetected hair tourniquet of a toe is part of the evaluation of unexplained pediatric crying. Bony injuries include FXs or dislocations. Most FXs of the toes and nondisplaced FXs of the metatarsals are not clinically significant. However, intra-articular, displaced, and multiple metatarsal FXs require prompt referral. Midfoot injuries should be evaluated for **Lisfranc sprain** or **fracture**. Nondisplaced **avulsion FX** of fifth metatarsal tuberosity requires only supportive measures. FX of the proximal fifth metatarsal 1.5 cm distal to the base of the tuberosity (**Jones** or **Dancer FX**) needs aggressive management because of risk of nonunion and avascular necrosis. Soft tissue infections range from **ingrown toenails** to **diabetic ulcers**, a serious complication usually requiring hospitalization. Spontaneous pain, with swelling and erythema of first MTPJ suggests gout (podagra).

MANAGEMENT

- Ice, elevation, NSAIDs, analgesia. Buddy tape toe FX, rigid ortho shoe, posterior mold, crutches. Orthopedic consult for unstable or clinically significant FX. Ingrown toenail: warm soaks, NSAIDs, BX, definitive toenail avulsion
- **Diabetic Ulcer Infection:** saline dressing, possible debridement, control hyperglycemia, consider **cellulitis** or x-ray to R/O **osteomyelitis**. Vancomycin 20 mg/kg IV BID plus ampicillin/sulbactam 3 g IV or piperacillin/tazobactam 4.5 g IV QID
- **Gout:** consider septic joint. NSAIDs, including indomethacin, analgesia, steroids, avoid alcohol and high-purine foods. Colchicine 1.2 mg PO, followed by 0.6 mg in 1 hour (review renal/hepatic function and recent meds for contraindications)

FOOT PAIN

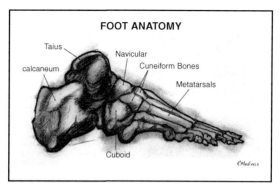

FOOT ANATOMY

Taius
Navicular
calcaneum
Cuneiform Bones
Metatarsals
Cuboid
R.Medina.s

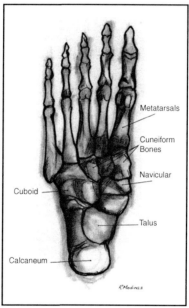

Metatarsals

Cuneiform Bones

Navicular

Cuboid

Talus

Calcaneum

R.Medina.s

DICTATION/DOCUMENTATION

- **General:** level of distress
- **VS and SaO$_2$** (if indicated)
- **Foot/Toes:** pt is able to bear weight and ambulate without pain. No surface trauma, ecchymosis, erythema, lesions, ulcers or break in skin integrity. The R/L foot is with/ without obvious asymmetry or deformity when compared to the R/L foot. No bony step-off, NT to palpation over toes, midfoot, or hind foot, or sole. Normal plantar/ dorsiflexion, inversion/eversion. Distal motor and neurovascular status are intact

FOOT PAIN

X-RAY NOTE: There was no fracture, dislocation, soft tissue swelling or FB noted.

SPLINT NOTE: There was no neurovascular compromise after splint/boot application; the splint/boot was in good alignment and the pt had good sensation and cap refill at the time of discharge.

ANKLE/FOOT X-RAY ORDERING CRITERIA:
- **Ankle X-Ray** should be ordered if malleolar zone pain and any of the following:
  - Age 55 or older
  - PT at posterior edge or tip of lateral malleolus, PT at posterior edge or tip of medial malleolus.

- **Foot X-Ray** should be ordered if there is any pain in the midfoot zone and any of the following:
  - Age 55 or older
  - PT at navicular and/or base of fifth metatarsal
  - Inability to bear weight both immediately and in the ED

Adapted from Perry, J. J., & Stiell, I. G. (2006). Impact of clinical decision rules on clinical care of traumatic injuries to the foot and ankle, knee, cervical spine, and head. *Injury*, *37*(12), 1157–1165.

⚙TIP
If unable to bear weight—crutches, then recheck 1 to 2 days

DON'T MISS!
- Lisfranc fracture
- Diabetic foot ulcer
- Vascular occlusion
- Hair tourniquet in infants/children

CHILD WITH LIMP

AGES 1 to 3

- **Minor Trauma:** most common, such as contusion, sprain, wound, or lesion on foot, hair tourniquet. Fractures less common; consider abuse
- **Transient Toxic Synovitis:** inability to bear weight due to pain caused by transient inflammation of synovium of hip joint. Common cause of unilateral nontraumatic hip or groin pain; may be referred to thigh or knee. Well-appearing child with recent viral infection in most cases; may have low-grade fever. Holds hip flexed with slight abduction and external rotation. Pain with gentle log rolling of leg is significant. Usually self-limiting and responds to analgesia. Consider septic arthritis or osteomyelitis. Full exam needed to identify viral causes, back pain (diskitis), abd etiology (appendicitis), GU (hernia, torsion) or other injuries. For new-onset limp in well child, diagnostic tests are often deferred to watchful waiting and follow-up in 24 hours. Possible CBC, ESR, CRP, UA; bilateral hip x-rays with frog view
- **Septic Arthritis:** orthopedic emergency than can lead to permanent damage. Usually febrile, ill-appearing child with inability to bear weight. Monoarticular—hip or knee most common. Joint is tender, red, warm, with decreased and painful ROM; swelling of hip can be difficult to assess. Hip flexed, abducted, and externally rotated; knee held in flexion. Diagnostics include CBC, ESR (>40), CRP, blood culture, arthrocentesis, x-rays or other imaging
- **Osteomyelitis:** acute bone infection often spread by bacteria from bloodstream. Often high fever, irritable, malaise, poor intake, decreased and painful ROM. Joint erythema, swelling, tenderness

AGES 4 to 10

- **Fractures:** more common—minor strain, contusion
- **Transient Toxic Synovitis:** possible until about age 10 years
- **Legg–Calve–Perthes Disease:** [also called avascular necrosis of femoral head (AVN)] collapse of hip joint and deformity of femoral head. More common in boys, 4:1. Achy pain in hip, groin, or back of knee; painful ROM of hip especially internal rotation and abduction. X-rays show small, flattened, fragmented femoral head
- **Cancer:** leukemia, osteosarcoma
- **Diskitis:** inflammatory Dx of intervertebral disk space. Pain radiates to legs, limp, unable to bear weight. Spine very tender to palpation

AGES 11 to TEENS

- **Trauma:** commonly caused by sports, MCV, assault
- **Osgood–Schlatter Disease:** benign, self-limiting pain and edema of tibial tubercle; outside knee joint; no effusion. More common in active boys during rapid growth. Usually unilateral; pain, swelling, tenderness just below patella. Improves with rest; exacerbated by jumping, kneeling, squatting, using stairs
- **Slipped Capital Femoral Epiphysis (SCFE):** posterior slip of femoral head from its neck at weak growth plate; more common in boys, Blacks, obese. Sudden or gradual onset. Holds leg in external rotation and has pain with internal rotation. Pain in hip, medial thigh, or referred only to knee. External rotation when trying to flex hip. AP/lateral/frog-leg x-rays; lateral femoral neck line (Klein's line) will not cross femoral head; wide, irregular physis
- Also consider: **gonococcal arthritis, HSP, sickle cell Dx, SLE, RA, malignancy, intra-abd or GU causes, abuse**

CHILD WITH LIMP

MDM/DDx

Children with limp often have undetected minor trauma, such as **contusions, sprains**, or **infection, such as ingrown toenails. Accidental physeal fracture** or **intentional abuse** must be considered. The history of recent viral illness supports the common etiology of **viral synovitis**. More serious causes of pediatric limp are **osteomyelitis, septic arthritis, bacterial synovitis**, or **diskitis**. Less common are **AVN, malignancy, RA**, or **intra-abd causes**.

MANAGEMENT

- Possible trauma = immobilize, x-ray, analgesia
- No trauma/not sick + pain = analgesia, re-examine, x-ray, consider septic joint, SCFE or AVN
- No trauma/"sick" + pain = pain/fever control, x-ray, CBC, ESR, CRP, blood cxs
- Consider joint aspiration, MRI

DICTATION/DOCUMENTATION

- **General:** level of distress
- **VS and SaO$_2$**
- **Lower Extremities:** there is/is no obvious asymmetry or deformity of the R/L leg when compared to the R/L leg. No surface trauma, ecchymosis, erythema, lesions, ulcers noted, including sole of foot. No bony step-off or deformity, NT to palpation of leg. Normal flexion/extension, abduction/adduction, internal and external log roll of hip. Knee is NT, FROM, no STS or effusion, popliteal fossa NT without swelling. Ankle, foot, and toes are NT with normal FROM. Gait is antalgic/Trendelenberg/waddling/stiff-legged/toe walking/steppage/slow. Distal motor and neurovascular status is intact. Include Abd, back, groin, GU exam

X-RAY NOTE: There was no fracture, dislocation, soft tissue swelling or FB noted.

SPLINT NOTE: There was no neurovascular compromise after splint application; the splint was in good alignment and the pt had good sensation and capillary refill at the time of discharge.

SALTER HARRIS GROWTH PLATE FRACTURES

SALTR

I   S = Same/Straight
II A = Above
III L = Lower
IV T = Through
V   R = Rammed/Crushed

MEB

M   Metaphysis
E   Epiphysis
B   Both

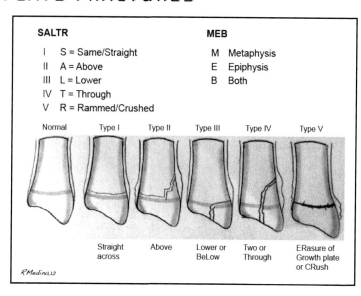

Normal	Type I	Type II	Type III	Type IV	Type V
	Straight across	Above	Lower or BeLow	Two or Through	ERasure of Growth plate or CRush

R Medina 12

LACERATIONS/PUNCTURE WOUNDS

HX
- Exact time of injury/delayed presentation/prior treatment
- MOI: blunt, penetrating, crush injury, organic matter, animal bite, FB
- Dominant hand, occupation, work related
- Puncture wound through tennis shoe (*Pseudomonas*)
- Contaminated with sea water
- High pressure paint gun, staple gun
- Closed fist wounds, fight bite
- Associated injury, self-inflicted wounds
- HX: Comorbidities: DM, immunosuppressed
- Meds/Allergies/Immunizations (Tetanus status)

PE
- **General:** level of distress, pain, F/C
- **VS and SaO$_2$**
- **Skin:** wound location, length, depth, linear, curvilinear, stellate, flap, jagged
    - Tissue loss, devitalized tissue, visible or palpable FB
    - Crush injury, exposed bone or tendon, active bleeding, STS, ecchymosis
    - Distal motor neurovascular status intact
    - Repeat motor exam under anesthesia and ROM
- **Note:** detailed motor neurovascular exam if injury to digit/extremity

MDM/DDx
Wounds are divided into types of repair: **simple, intermediate, or complex.** Anatomic location and wound length in centimeters must also be noted. Multiple wounds can be reported in total centimeters unless the wounds are of varying complexity. **Simple repair** includes closure of superficial wounds involving only the skin, regardless of length. Intermediate lacerations include approximation of skin and subcutaneous layer, galia, or superficial fascia. Simple wound closure that required extensive cleaning and removal of particulate matter may be classified as intermediate in some cases. **Complex repair** includes multiple layer repair, debridement, extensive undermining, or placement of retention sutures.

MANAGEMENT
- Thorough wound irrigation and exploration with adequate hemostasis is the foundation of wound care. Identification of underlying deep structure injury or retained FB is essential for optimal wound healing.
- Wounds that may require specialty referral include:
    - Large avulsions or near amputations
    - Severe crush injuries and/or devitalized tissue involvement of eyelid tarsal plate or tear duct system; auricular hematoma
    - Large cartilage defects
- X-ray for FB may be indicated. Tetanus: Adults >19 yrs, substitute 1-time dose of Tdap for Td booster; then boost with Td every 10 yrs
- Consider ABX for contaminated wounds, delayed presentation, older adults or immunosuppressed pts

LACERATIONS/PUNCTURE WOUNDS

SUTURE REMOVAL
- 4 to 5 days: eyelid, lip, face
- 4 to 6 days: pinna ear, neck
- 7 days: scalp/head
- 10 to 12 days: trunk or extremity
- 12 to 14 days: hand or foot—unless child (may be less days)
- If wound is healing poorly or infected, consider retained FB

SUTURE SIZE
- 6.0 Face
- 5.0 Hand
- 4.0 Extrems

LACERATION PROCEDURE NOTE: The procedure was explained and consent obtained. The wound was anesthetized with _____ mL of _____ with good anesthesia. (Note local infiltration, field block, digital block.) Sterile drape and prep were done. Copious irrigation was done with saline and the wound explored. (Note whether able to visualize depth of wound.) There was no FB or deep structure injury noted. (Note whether examined under range of motion.) Wound edges were approximated with good alignment using_____ (sutures, staples, skin adhesive, skin tapes.) There were (number) of sutures/staples placed with_____type of suture. Type of dressing applied, if done. The pt tolerated the procedure well without adverse effects.

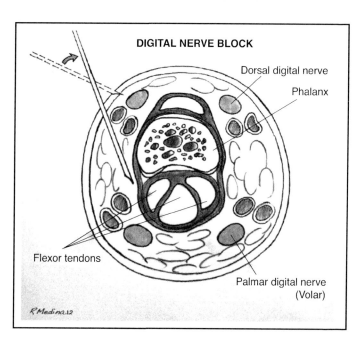

DIGITAL NERVE BLOCK

Dorsal digital nerve

Phalanx

Flexor tendons

Palmar digital nerve (Volar)

R.Medina.12

LACERATIONS/PUNCTURE WOUNDS

DON'T MISS!

- Advise pt of possible retained FB—note in chart
- Open fracture, tendon injury, joint capsule disruption, neurovascular dysfunction

ABSCESS/CELLULITIS

HX
- Onset, duration
- F/C, N/V
- Injury, insect, animal (e.g., dog, cat), human bite, FB, illicit drug use
- History or exposure to complicated skin infections (MRSA)
- MRSA risk factors
- Current treatment
- Tetanus status
- Comorbidities: immunosuppressed (DM, Hep C, HIV), alcoholic, recent post op wound

PE
- **General:** F/C, malaise
- **VS and SaO$_2$**
- **Skin:**
    - Localized pain/tenderness, swelling, erythema, fluctuance, induration
    - Pointing, drainage, palpable crepitus
    - Central eschar formation
    - Surrounding erythema, warmth
    - Proximal lymphangitis, regional lymphadenopathy
    - Distal edema
- Describe location, size, shape, consistency, margins
- Perform rectal exam if in perianal area—note fissures, tenderness, mass, fluctuance

MDM/DDx
Small abscesses without cellulitis usually require only simple incision and drainage followed by supportive measures such as warm soaks. Midface infections are at risk for **carvernous sinus thrombosis. Extensive** or **multiple abscesses**, especially in immunocompromised pts, are clinically significant. **Perianal abscesses** are areas of concern because it is difficult to determine the extent of abscess formation and can lead to fistula formation. Other abscesses are caused by **hidradenitis suppurativa**, infected **sebaceous cysts, pilonidal cyst**, or **staph infections**. Consider infected lymph node vs. abscess formation on neck or groin areas. **Erysipelas** is a cellulitis that causes a painful, very red plaque with raised and sharply defined borders. Small areas of cellulitis without necrosis often improve with only a short course of oral antibiotics. Complex situations include large or **rapidly spreading cellulitis, failed outpatient treatment, immunosuppression**, or **signs of sepsis**. The very young, old, and **debilitated** are at risk for rapid deterioration from infection. Severe soft tissue infections may result in **necrotizing fasciitis** (rapidly spreading cellulitis with ulcers, necrosis, crepitus, bullae). Periorbital cellulitis (preseptal) must be evaluated for extension to **orbital cellulitis**. Erysipelas caused by group A beta-hemolytic streptococci is a painful infection that causes an area of erythema and swelling with a sharply demarcated border; usually on the legs or face.

MANAGEMENT
- Adequate I&D is foundation of treatment
- Packing: none or wick only to keep wound open
- Warm soaks, NSAIDs
- ABX not usually indicated unless immunosuppressed, DM, MRSA, multiple abscesses, cellulitis
- Consult for perirectal abscess

ABSCESS/CELLULITIS

MANAGEMENT CELLULITIS
- Consider hyperglycemia
- Fever control, NSAIDs, analgesia, elevation, and warm soaks
- Possible soft tissue x-ray or Ultz to R/O FB or gas
- ABX (7–10 days): clindamycin 450 mg TID; doxycycline 100 mg PO BID; TMP/SMX (DS) 1 to 2 tabs PO BID; amoxicillin/clavulanate 875 mg PO BID; cephalexin 500 mg PO QID; dicloxacillin 500 mg PO QID; Vancomycin 15 to 20 mg/kg IV QID; clindamycin 600 mg IV TID
- Tetanus: Adults >19 yrs, substitute 1-time dose of Tdap for Td booster; then boost with Td every 10 yrs
- **Erysipelas:** azithromycin 500 mg PO × 1 then 250 mg daily × 4 days; 10 days course for other ABX, for example, dicloxacillin 500 mg PO QID; cephalexin 500 mg PO QID; clindamycin 450 mg PO TID
- Recheck 1 to 2 days, sooner if worse
- Admit for IV ABX if immunosuppressed, extensive, rapid spread, failed outpatient, toxic

ABSCESS I&D PROCEDURE NOTE: The procedure was explained and consent obtained. The wound was anesthetized with _____ mL of _____ with good anesthesia. Sterile drape and prep were done. The fluctuant center was incised with #11 blade scalpel. A small/moderate/large amount of (exudate/blood/caseous material) was expressed or removed. The wound was probed for loculated areas and irrigated with normal saline. Note whether the wound was packed loosely with wick or left open. DSD was applied. The pt tolerated the procedure well.

DON'T MISS!
- Extensive or circumferential cellulitis with severe pain
- Necrotizing fasciitis—rapidly spreading erythema and pain within hours
- Orbital cellulitis
- Hand cellulitis

INDEX